PHARMACOLOGY - RESEARCH, SAFETY TESTING AND REGULATION

SIMVASTATIN DELIVERY

CHALLENGES AND OPPORTUNITIES

PHARMACOLOGY - RESEARCH, SAFETY TESTING AND REGULATION

Additional books in this series can be found on Nova's website under the Series tab.

Additional e-books in this series can be found on Nova's website under the e-book tab.

PHARMACOLOGY - RESEARCH, SAFETY TESTING AND REGULATION

SIMVASTATIN DELIVERY

CHALLENGES AND OPPORTUNITIES

ALBERTO A. C. C. PAIS
JOÃO J. S. SOUSA
AND
CARLA VITORINO
EDITORS

NOVA BIOMEDICAL

New York

Additional color graphics may be available in the e-book version of this book.

Library of Congress Cataloging-in-Publication Data

ISBN: 978-1-63482-148-3
Library of Congress Control Number: 2015931780

Published by Nova Science Publishers, Inc. † New York

Contents

Preface

Statins are the most commonly prescribed drugs for the treatment of dyslipidemia or related diseases, being considered of superior effectiveness for that purpose. Simvastatin (SV), one of the most important drugs within the statins class, is a potent inhibitor of the enzyme 3-hydroxy-3-methylglutaryl coenzyme A reductase, involved in the cholesterol synthesis. This inhibition is mainly responsible for reducing low density lipoprotein (LDL, usually considered the "bad cholesterol") levels, but it has also been shown to reduce the levels of triglycerides and increase those of high density lipoprotein, HDL ("good cholesterol"). It has also been reported as effective in the reduction of the morbidity and mortality associated to the coronary heart disease. Now, millions of patients benefit from the use of simvastatin in preventing coronary heart disease.

Recently, SV has been identified as a multifaceted drug, addressing different physiological and pathological conditions, thus extending beyond the conventional cholesterol-dependent mechanisms. It has triggered the development of new strategies in order to promote the respective delivery through novel routes of administration. Combined regimens of simvastatin with different drugs with noteworthy health benefits in the concomitant treatment of several conditions have also been considered in recent developments.

In this book, a comprehensive selection of topics is presented, encompassing aspects that firstly include chemical synthesis and pharmacology.

The chemical synthesis is addressed from a historical perspective, also focusing on relevant issues, such as "green chemistry" and recent developments. The pharmacology of SV is treated with particular emphasis on new therapeutic applications.

In a second part, several delivery systems for new therapeutic areas are explored. These comprise nanoemulsions administered through the parenteral route, nanostructured lipid carriers for transdermal delivery and supramolecular systems for a local application. Cancer therapy and bone regeneration are some of the therapeutic targets addressed along with the classical treatment of hypercholesterolemia, now in drug combination therapies.

Delivery systems based on nanoemulsions and related systems are increasingly being utilized in the pharmaceutical industry to deliver lipophilic bioactive compounds, such as simvastatin. The small size of the particles in this kind of delivery systems (< 100 nm) means that they have a number of potential benefits for certain applications: enhanced long-term stability; high optical clarity; and, increased bioavailability. Parenteral lipid nanoemulsions are also a novel platform for the delivery of simvastatin for subsequent use in combination chemotherapy, and to evaluate the respective antiproliferative activity.

Lipid nanoparticles or, more specifically, nanostructured lipid carriers (NLC), are colloidal systems, made of a blend of liquid and solid lipids, stabilized in an aqueous surfactant(s) solution. NLC claim several advantages for improving penetration of drugs, in particular SV, through the skin. These include their chemical similarity to skin lipids, stemming from the common hydrophobic character, the existence of a solid matrix, and the biocompatibility, which make these carriers suitable for long-term controlled-release skin administration.

Some studies about the positive effect of simvastatin on bone tissue have been confirmed both *in vitro* and *in vivo*. In local delivery, the effects of simvastatin on osteoblast differentiation were promoted by their anabolic activity on bone through the promotion of osteoblasts differentiation. Compared to other synthetic osteoinductive agents, simvastatin offers additional benefits, such as promotion of new blood vessel growth. Simvastatin can stimulate high expression of bone morphogenetic protein (BMP)-2 in osteoblasts, and can effectively stimulate bone matrix formation. In this sense, supramolecular polymer chemistry has emerged as a fascinating subject within macromolecular research. Supramolecular structures involving macrocyclic compounds have attracted tremendous interest not only as models for understanding natural supramolecular self-assembly and molecular recognition, but also as precursors for designing novel nanomaterials for electronics, biomedical and pharmaceutical application and targeted delivery of therapeutic agents or bioactive materials.

This book benefits from the participation of recognized experts from different areas. These include researchers from pharmaceutical technology, pharmacology and synthetic chemistry.

In: Simvastatin Delivery
Editors: Alberto A. C. C. Pais et al.
ISBN: 978-1-63482-148-3

Chapter 1

Synthesis of Simvastatin: Historical Perspective and New Developments

Marta Pineiro[*]
Department of Chemistry, University of Coimbra, Coimbra, Portugal

Abstract

Simvastatin is one of the best selling drugs worldwide, requiring the production of a huge amount of this drug, which has driven the search for simple, cheap and environmentally friendly methods of synthesis that allow the preparation of simvastatin with the least possible amount of impurities. This chapter reviews the methods of preparation of simvastatin, from the earliest synthetic ones, patented by Merck, to the last innovations using biocatalysts.

Keywords: Simvastin synthesys, biocatalysis, semi-synthetic routes, sequential acylation

* Department of Chemistry, University of Coimbra, Rua Larga, 3004-535 Coimbra, Portugal Email: mpineiro@qui.uc.pt

Introduction

Aspergillus terreus is a worldwide distributed fungus that can be found in a variety of habitats, including warm soil, compost or dust. It is responsible for causing diseases such as allergic bronchopulmonary aspergillosis, aspergillus bronchitis and invasive aspergillus tracheobronchitis, invasive (pulmonary) aspergillosis and disseminated aspergillosis. Also, and not less important it is the original source of lovastatin (1), [1-2] a fungal metabolite, and important organic acids such as itaconic (2) acid and cis-aconitic acid (3), Figure 3, as well as commercially important enzymes that include xylanase.

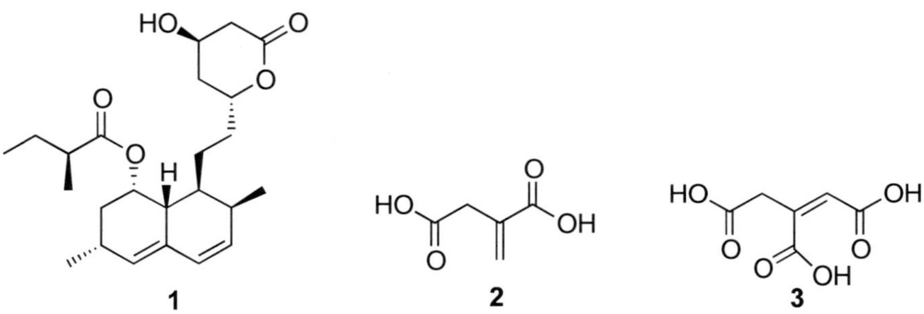

Figure 1. Structure of organic compounds isolated from Aspergillus terreus.

Lovastatin (mevinolin) (1) represents the first of a new class of hypolipidemic agents (HMG CoA reductase inhibitors) that are used to lower the levels of cholesterol in the body. Lovastatin is the precursor for the synthesis of a more active hypolipaemic agent (1S,3R,7S,8S,8aR)-8-(2-((2R,4R)-4-hydroxy-6-oxotetrahydro-2*H*-pyran-2-yl)ethyl)-3, 7-dimethyl-1,2,3,7,8,8a-hexahydronaphthalen-1-yl 2,2-dimethylbutanoate, also known as synvinolin or, more frequently, named simvastatin (4), Figure 2. The similarity in the structures of lovastatin and simvastatin is evident; they only differ in the additional methyl group at position 2 of the butyrate ester substituent. Thus, the simplest route to obtain simvastatin should be a simple alkylation reaction. However, it has been reported that the direct alkylation is not a viable process because the higher acidity of the lactone α-H when compared with the α-H atoms of the ester chain leads to products with the alkyl group at the lactone moiety. [3] In fact, the attempts of direct methylation of lovastatin resulted in poor conversion coupled with many side reactions, which complicates both isolation and purification of the final product.[4] Therefore, the synthesis of simvastatin from lovastatin is a more complex process.

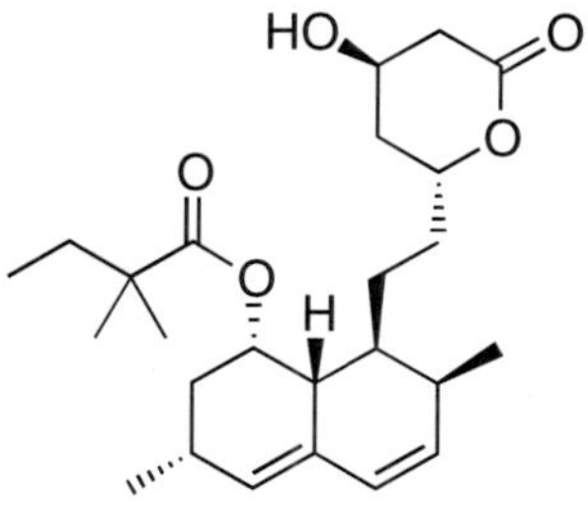

4

Figure 2. Simvastatin structure.

Semi-Synthetic Routes to Simvastatin

The transformation of lovastatin into simvastatin could be achieved through two main routes drafted in Figure 3, one (blue) requires protection of the lactone moiety, methylation and deprotection and the other (orange) comprises a deacylation process, removing the 2-methylbutyryl group on the naphthalene moiety, and forming a derivative with two hydroxyl groups; consequently, before acylation with 2,2-dimethylbutyryl chloride the hydroxyl group at the lactone ring must be protected.

The methodology to transform lovastatin into simvastatin was first described by William F. Hoffman, Robert L. Smith and Alvin K. Willard and patented in 1984. [5] During the period of approval (the patent was filed in 1980) Smith and Willard published a detailed procedure while they studied process for the incorporation of ^{14}C into the lovastatin structure. [6] Treatment of lovastatin with lithium hydroxide in water at reflux resulted in the rapid opening of the lactone ring followed by slow hydrolysis of the 2-methylester. The cyclization to recover the lactone ring was achieved after neutralization and heating at toluene reflux during two hours with a Dean-Stark apparatus for azeotropic removal of water. The hydroxyl derivative **5**, with the same stereochemical characteristics as lovastatin was obtained in 76% yield. Selective protection of the lactone hydroxyl **5** was accomplished by treatment with *tert*-butyldimethylchlorosilane **6** and imidazole in *N,N*-dimethylformamide (DMF) at 20 ºC for 18 h and after work-up the silyl ether **7** was obtained with 69% yield, Scheme 1.

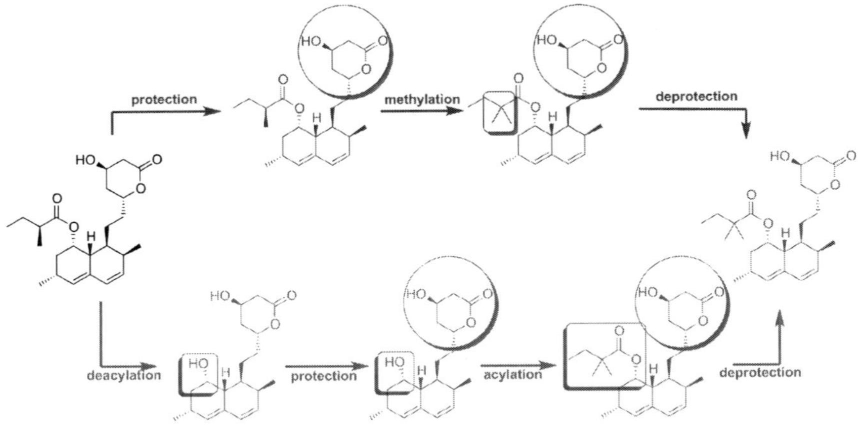

Figure 3. Methylation route (blue) and acylation route (orange) to obtain simvastatin from lovastatin.

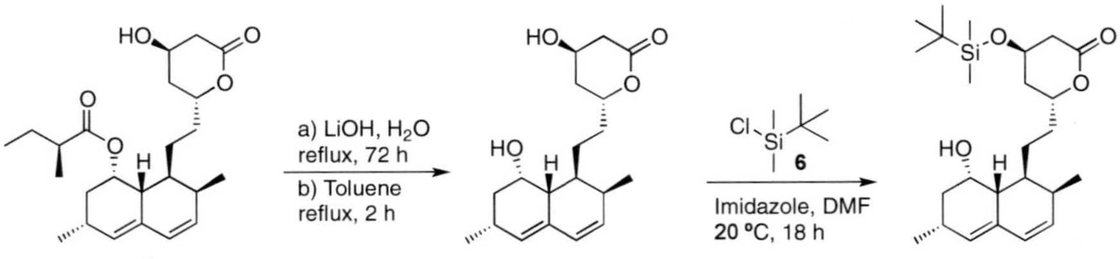

Scheme 1. Deacylation and protection of **1** with *tert*-butyldimethylchlorosilane.

The authors also described a method for the acylation of the protected alcohol **7** using a mixture of 4-dimethylaminopyridine (DMAP) and pyridine as solvent and 2-methylbutyrylchloride labeled with ^{14}C, followed by deprotection of the silyl derivative with tetrabutlyammonium fluoride trihydrate in THF. However, only in 1986, jointly with W.F. Hoffman and other coworkers, did they describe the synthesis of 21 side chain ester derivatives of lovastatin, including simvastatin, based on this methodology. [7] Simvastatin was synthetized from the reaction of silyl ether **7** with 2,2-dimethylbutyryl chloride **8** (previously prepared by heating the corresponding acid and 2 equiv of thionyl chloride at 100 °C for 2 h) in pyridine containing DMAP or 4-pyrrolidinopyridine as catalysts, heated at 100 °C under a N_2 atmosphere for 18 h. These harsh conditions for the acylation reaction were needed in the case of more hindered alkyl chlorides such as 2,2-

dimethylbutyryl chloride. As an alternative, the acylation of alcohol **7** was also achieved using acyl chloride **8** and LiBr in pyridine. [8] Deprotection of the silyl ether **9** was achieved with tetrabutylammonium fluoride trihydrate in THF and acetic acid at room temperature during 18 h; the use of acetic acid allows the attenuation of the basicity of fluoride avoiding the destruction of the lactone ring, Scheme 2. Also, simvastatin could be prepared in a four-step methodology involving: de-esterification of 2-methylbutyrate, protection of the 4-hydroxy group of the lactone ring, re-esterification of the side chain with 2,2-dimethylbutyrate (**8**) and deprotection of the 4-hydroxy group with an overall yield of 48%.

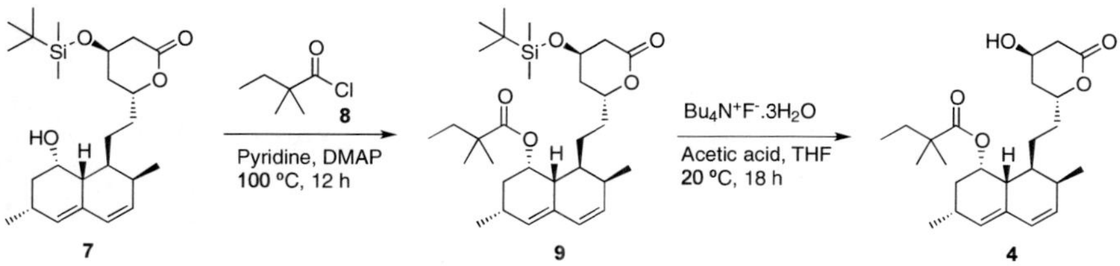

Scheme 2. Acylation of **7** with 2,2-dimethylbutyryl chloride followed by deprotection of the silyl derivative.

The introduction of simvastatin in the market led to the need for high-yielding, economical and environmentally acceptable processes. The main identified problems of the transformation of lovastatin to simvastatin are the contamination of simvastatin with the starting material lovastatin, which is very difficult to eliminate by fractional crystallization or column chromatography (USP limit of **1** in **4** is <1%), the large number of steps involved and the high costs of reagents. To solve these problems constituted the driving force for the development of new processes. Therefore, new methodologies to achieve the large–scale synthesis of simvastatin with less than 0.5% of lovastatin were developed. One of these methodologies involves the opening of the lactone ring through the preparation of amide **10** by heating lovastatin and butylamine at 80 °C for 1 h with quantitative yield. The crude amide **10** reacts with *tert*-butyldimethylsilyl chloride (TBSCl) **6** in DMF at 60°C for 6 h yielding the protected derivative **11** with 99% yield determined by HPLC assay. The reaction of derivative **11** with lithium pyrrolidine, prepared from pyrrolidine and *n*-butyl lithium, followed by quenching with 1.5 equivalents of methyl iodide gave extremely high conversions into the methylated derivatives **12a** and **12b** (99.7%) with a **12a/12b** ratio of 30. Acid-catalyzed silyl transfer with methanesulfonic acid in aqueous methanol at 30

°C for 5 h afforded the dihydroxyamides **13a** and **13b**. The addition of sodium hydroxide to the desilylation reaction crude, followed by heating and collection of the distillate (vapor temperature 72-73 °C) at ambient pressure, resulted in the complete amide hydrolysis. The reaction product was efficiently isolated as the highly crystalline ammonium salt derivative **14** after reaction with a solution of aqueous ammonium hydroxide in methanol. Lactonization to afford simvastatin (**4**) was achieved with 94.2% yield by heating de ammonium salt in toluene at 100 °C for 6 h, Scheme 3. [9] The overall yield for the transformation from lovastatin to simvastatin, comprising six steps, was 86%.

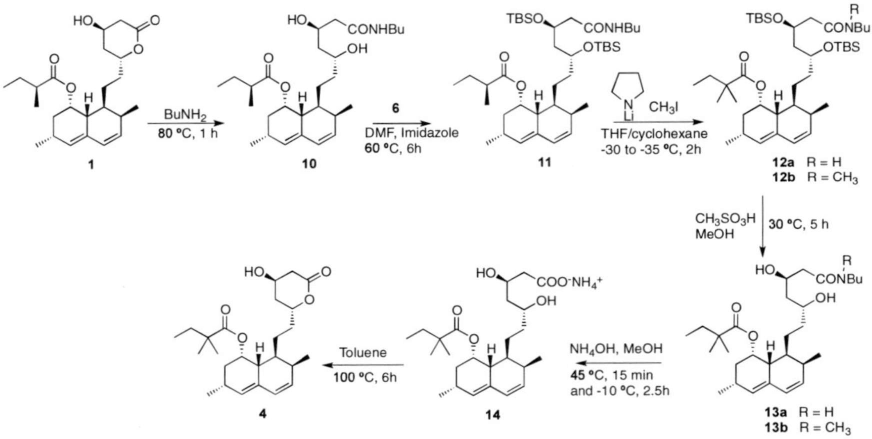

Scheme 3. Synthesis of simvastatin through methylation and using primary amines.

In an effort to reduce the number of steps needed, Thaper and co-workers reported a cost-efficient synthesis of simvastatin involving four steps, eliminating two expensive chemical protection and deprotection steps of the open dihydroxyacid form. [10] The reaction of lovastatin (**1**) with excess cyclopropylamine (**15**) at 42 °C for 6 h gave the corresponding amide **16** with quantitative yield. This amide can also be obtained by reaction of mevinolinic acid ammonium salt **18** with cyclopropylamine in toluene. The amide was methylated by means of BuLi, methyl iodide and pyrrolidine in THF at low temperature yielding the dimethylbutyryl derivative **17a** contaminated with only 2-3% of *N*-methylated derivative **17b**. Hydrolysis of **17** with NaOH in refluxing methanol, followed by treatment with NH_4OH in methanol affords the ammonium salt **14** with 97.6% yield, which is finally lactonized in toluene to yield, after workup, simvastatin as a white crystalline product with an overall yield, of 85% and a purity higher than 99% determined by HPLC, Scheme 4.

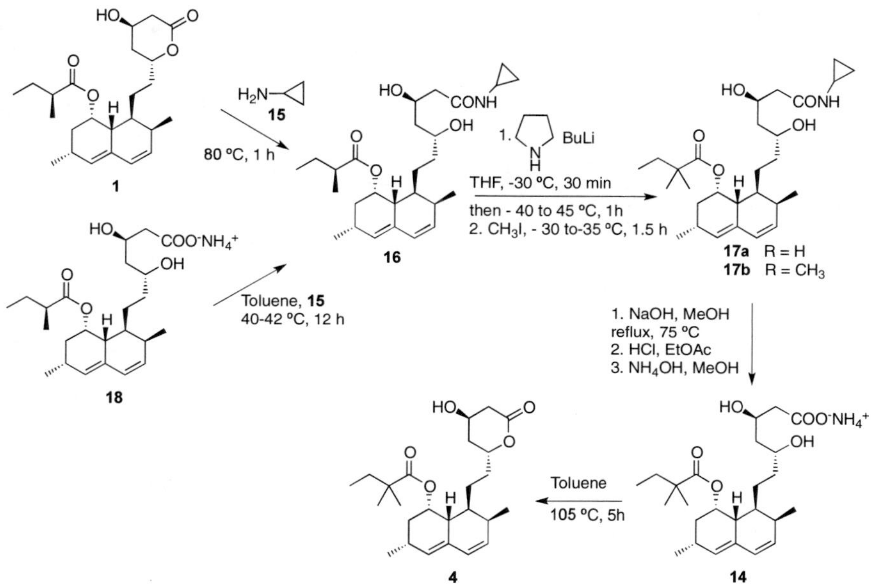

Scheme 4. Synthesis of simvastatin involving cyclopropylamine.

A different strategy comprising the sequential acylation of the diol lactone **5** to form a bis acylated intermediate followed by selective deacylation and lactonization, was developed by Debora and Tewalt in 1992. [11] The reaction of diol lactone **5** with acetic anhydride catalyzed by DMAP in dry pyridine at 0 °C for 4-6 hours affords the 4-acetylated derivative **19** which after work-up was acetylated again using similar conditions at 35-40 °C for 48 h and 2,2-dimethylbutyrate (**8**) instead of acetic anhydride giving the diacetilated derivative, 4-acetyl simvastatin **20**. The de-acetylation reaction with HCl and methanol affords, after 16 h of stirring at room temperature, simvastatin methyl ester **21** which was transformed into the simvastatin ammonium salt **14** by treatment with NaOH in water at room temperature for 1-2 hours followed by neutralization with HCl and treatment with ammonium hydroxide in methanol at 10 °C during 30 min. The lactonization reaction was achieved by dissolving the ammonium salt in acetic acid with butylated hydroxyanisole and stirring the solution at 20-25 °C for 2 hours, after the addition of methanesulfonic acid, Scheme 5. The reaction yields or the overall yield of this process are not mentioned, nonetheless, the purity of the final product was calculated as 98 % by HPLC assay.

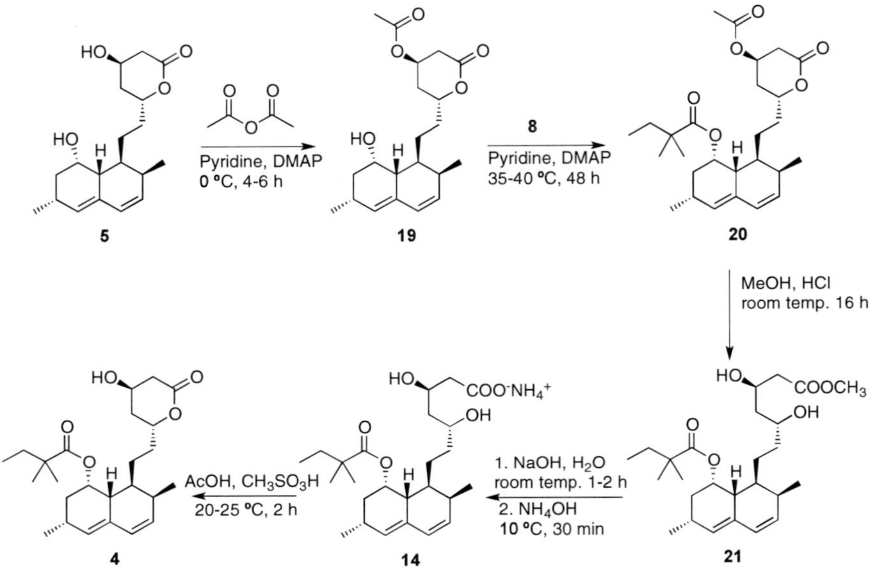

Scheme 5. Sequential acylation for the synthesis of simvastatin.

Two new related processes to synthesize simvastatin have been described based on the selective reduction of the carbonyl function of the lactone moiety of lovastatin to a hemiacetal. [12] The reduction of the lactone function of lovastatin with a solution of diisobutylaluminum hydride in dichloromethane slowly added to a solution of lovastatin in THF and stirred for 1 hour at -35 °C yields the hemiacetal **22** in 99% yield, with 96% purity. The hemiacetal reacts with acetyl chloride in methanol at room temperature for 15 min to afford acetal **23** with 98% yield and 95% purity. The methylation of the resulting acetal with methyl iodide using BuLi and pyrrolidine in THF affords the 2,2-dimethylbutyric acid ester **24** in 96% yield and 93% purity, which treated with diluted HCl in THF at room temperature for 1.5 h produces hemiacetal **25** quantitatively as a brown syrup with 75% purity. Finally, this compound is oxidized with Ag_2CO_3 in refluxing toluene for 2 h, protected from light, to afford simvastatin after work-up and crystallization from cyclohexane-heptane(l:l), in 48% yield, as a white solid. Alternatively, the direct methylation of hemiacetal **22** with methyl iodide by BuLi and pyrrolidine in

THF directly yields the methylated hemiacetal **25**, although with a slightly less purity, Scheme 6.

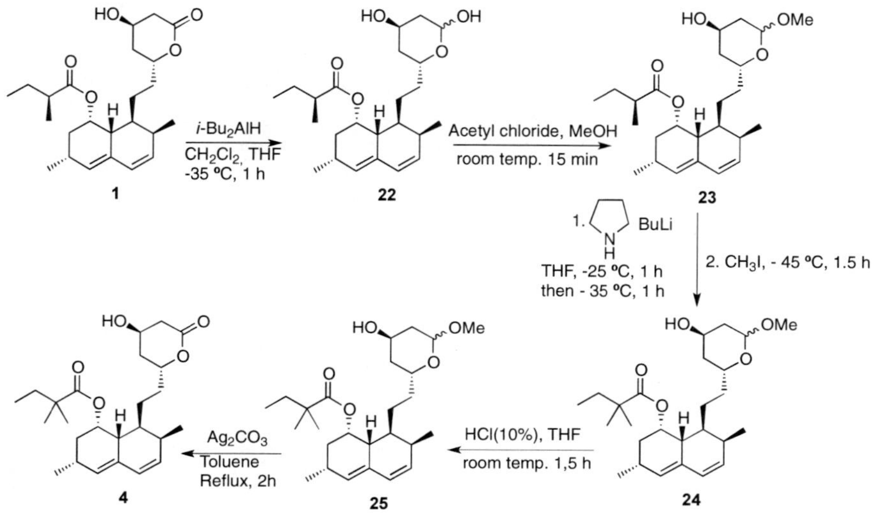

Scheme 6. Selective reduction of the carbonyl function of the lactone moiety of lovastatin for the synthesis of simvastatin.

The use of boronic acid as a protecting group of the hydroxyl group of lovastatin before methylation was also described as a methodology with some advantages for the industrial scale preparation of simvastatin. [13] The reaction of lovastatin with a primary amine, such as cyclohexylamine (**26**), in toluene at 110 ºC for 6 h results in the open chain derivative **27** that after work-up reacts with phenylboronic acid (**28**) in toluene at room temperature for 2 h to afford the protected derivative **29**. After the methylation of this boronate derivative, with methyliodine and lithium pyrrolidine in a similar manner as previously described, the hydroxyl groups were de-protected by passing a methanolic solution of **30**, through a column charged with activated Amberlite IRA-400 resin, developed with water-methanol (1:1) and eluted with methanol. The resulting dihydroxyamide **31** was transformed into simvastatin by lactonization catalyzed by acetic acid in a toluene-water biphasic system for 18 h, Scheme 7.

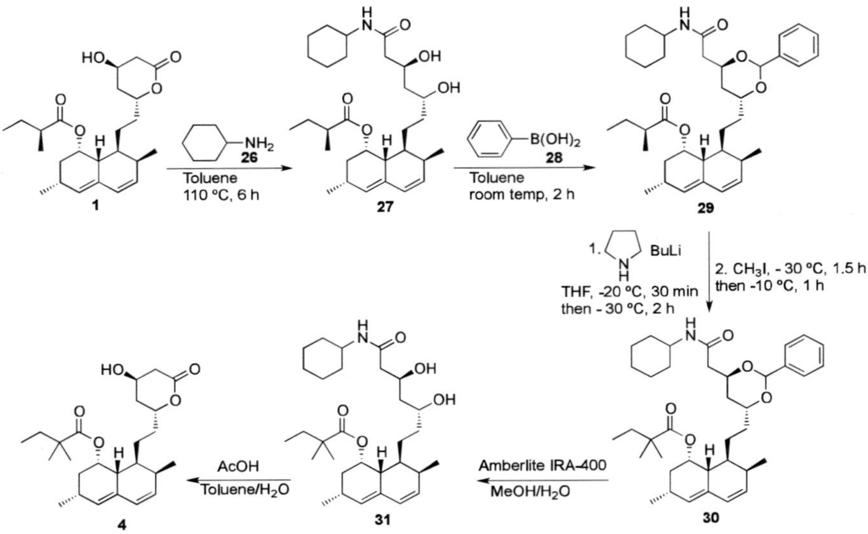

Scheme 7. Synthesis of simvastatin through the protection of amide derivatives with boronic acid.

Boronic acids were also used as protecting groups of the hydroxyl group at the lactone ring without previous formation of the amide derivative. [14] The hemiboronation of lovastatin was achieved by heating a equimolar suspension of lovastatin and phenylboronic acid (**28**) in toluene at 100-105 °C for 55 min. After work-up, the hemiphenylboronate **32** was obtained in 97% yield and 99% purity determined by HPLC. Once the methylation of this derivative using the established method with methyl iodide and lithium pyrrolidine was complete to yield 98.4% of the hemiphenylboronate derivative of simvastatin **33** at 95% purity by HPLC, the de-protection was accomplished by heating **33** and 1,3-propanediol or neopentyl glycol in toluene, giving simvastatin with 88% and 76% yield respectively, Scheme 8.

Already in the 21st century, Dabak and Adiyaman reported the use of ethylene glycol as a protecting group of the lactone carbonyl group to prevent alkylation at the α–position of the lactone ring.[15] Lovastatin (**1**) was transformed into the benzoate derivative **35** with benzylchoride (**34**) and pyridine in CH_2Cl_2, in 95% yield. The benzoate derivative was then treated with ethanediol **36**, triethyl ortoformate and a catalytic amount of sulfuric acid in THF as catalyst to afford protected benzoate **37** in 51% yield. Subsequent methylation using the established methodology with butyl lithium, pyrrolidine and methyl iodine, afforded protected simvastatin **38** in 85% yield. It is noteworthy that the deprotection of the hydroxyl group at the lactone ring occurs simultaneously in these reaction conditions. Removal of the protecting group by acid catalyzed hydrolysis at room temperature gave simvastatin in 92% yield, Scheme 9.

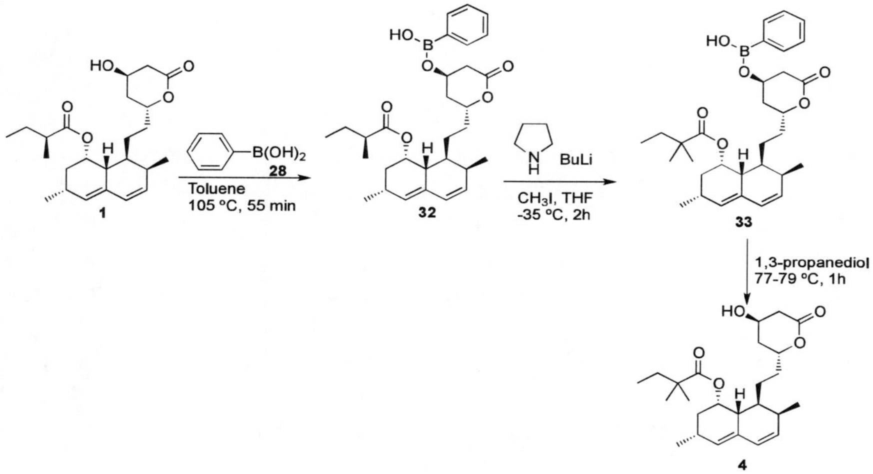

Scheme 8. Synthesis of simvastatin through the protection of the lactone ring with boronic acid.

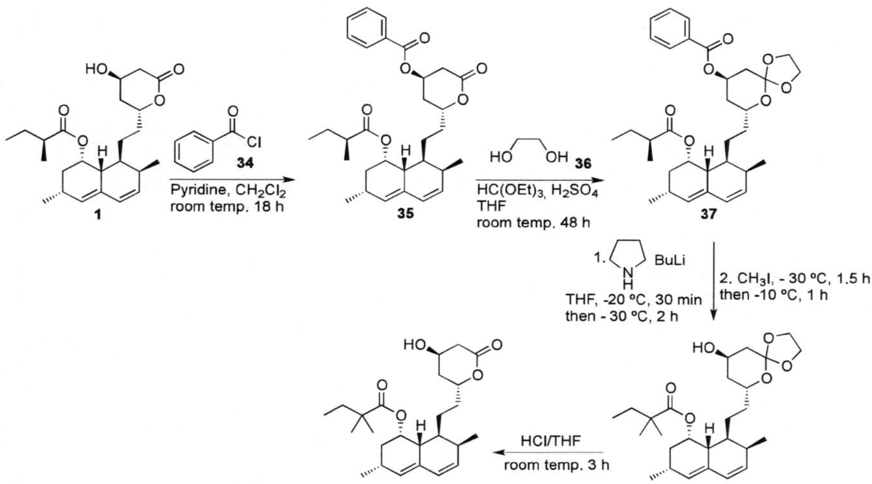

Scheme 9. Ethylene glycol as protecting group of the lactone carbonyl group for the synthesis of simvastatin.

The referred methods for the synthesis of simvastatin by treating lovastatin or the salt form of mevolinic acid with a primary amine avoiding the hydroxyl protection and deprotection sequence (see Scheme 4) presents as the main problem the formation of undesirable amounts of by-products due to the occurrence of side reactions at the amide group. For example, with methyl iodide, used in the methylation step, to yield *N*-methyl derivatives such as **17b**. To overcome this problem, secondary amines were used for the formation of the amide form of lovastatin. [16] Amide derivative **39** was obtained by reaction of lovastatin with diethyl amine in refluxing toluene for 36 h; derivatives **40** and **41** resulted from the reaction of cyclic secondary amines, pyrrolidine and piperidine respectively, without any additional solvent, in 5-6 h. Methylation of these amide derivatives affords secondary amides represented by **42**. Subsequent transformation into the ammonium salt and cyclization to form simvastatin were performed as previously described by introducing slight modifications such as the use of ethanol instead of methanol for the amide hydrolysis, and NH_3 gas instead of ammonium hydroxide for the formation of the ammonium salt **14**, Scheme 10. As in the original method, this strategy avoids the protection and deprotection of the hydroxyl groups at the heptyl chain.

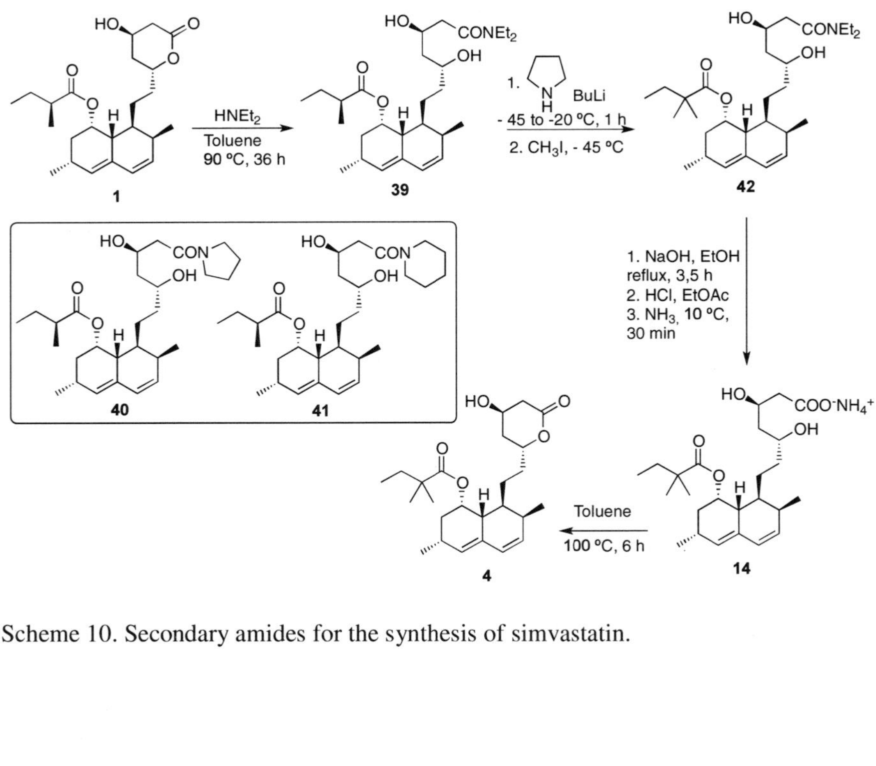

Scheme 10. Secondary amides for the synthesis of simvastatin.

Using as starting material the hydroxylsilyl derivative **7**, and seventeen years later, Kim and coworkers improved Hoffman original methodology, achieving the *in situ* esterification using 2,2-dimethylbutanoic acid (**43**) activated with triphenylphosphine and hexachloroethane in dichloromethane. [17] The reaction of 1-((chlorotriphenylphosphoranyl)oxy)-2,2-dimethylbutan-1-one (**44**) with the hydroxyl group of derivative **7** yields protected simvastatin almost quantitatively. Deprotection was carried out with methanesulfonic acid at 50 ºC for 3 h, Scheme 11.

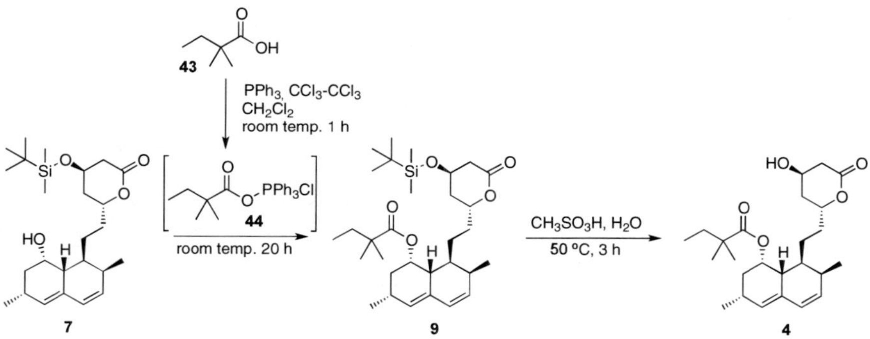

Scheme 11. Activation of 2,2-dimethylbutanoic acid by triphenylphosphine.

Another process designed to improved the acylation process, in this case avoiding the use of silyl derivatives as protectiving groups in order to increase the purity of the final products, suggest the use of ketones or acetals as protecting groups. [18]. Starting from lovastatin, deacylation and lactonization were achieved using KOH and *tert*-butyl alcohol followed by acidification with methanesulfonic acid in isopropyl acetate. The reaction of diol lactone **5** with 2,2-dimethoxypropene **45** in dicloromethane catalyzed by *p*-toluenesulfonic acid at room temperature for 1 h afforded the protected alcohol **46**. Following acylation using 2,2-dimethylbutyl chloride in pyridine and 4-dimethylaminopyridine at 100 ºC during 6 h gave the protected simvastatin **47** that was transformed into simvastatin by reaction with HCl in acetonitrile at room temperature for 4 h, Scheme 12.

The use of *N*-methylimidazol as solvent allows the improvement of the synthesis of simvastatin by acylation, combining in a single step the protection of the hydroxyl group on the lactone ring and the acylation reaction. As an additional advantage, the reaction temperature decreases when compared with other acylation reactions, increasing the purity of the final product [19], Scheme 13.

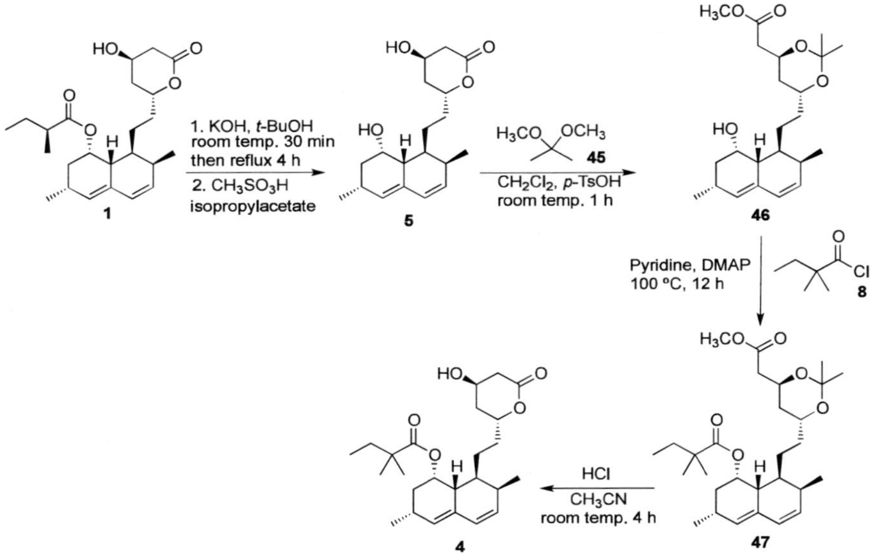

Scheme 12. The use of ketones or acetals as protecting groups in the synthesis of simvastatin.

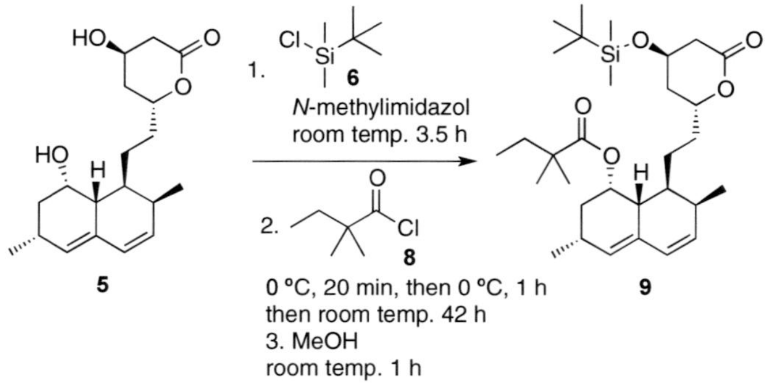

Scheme 13. One-step protection and acylation using *N*-methylimidazol.

More recently, and still looking for a more robust and scalable route to simvastatin incorporing methylation, 3,4-dihydro-2*H*-pyrane (**48**) was used as a cost-effective, nonhazardous and easy to handle protecting group. [20] The reaction of lovastatin with dihydropyrane **48** catalyzed by sulfuric acid affords the protected lovastatin **49** in 25 min which *in situ* reacts with butylamine to give the open chain derivative **50** almost quantitatively (without purification).

This derivative, with only one protected hydroxyl group was successfully methylated giving derivative **51**, transformed into the ammonium salt form **52** and cyclized using *p*-toluenesulfonic acid in a toluene/acetonitrile mixture to obtain simvastatin in 93% yield and 99% purity, Scheme 14.

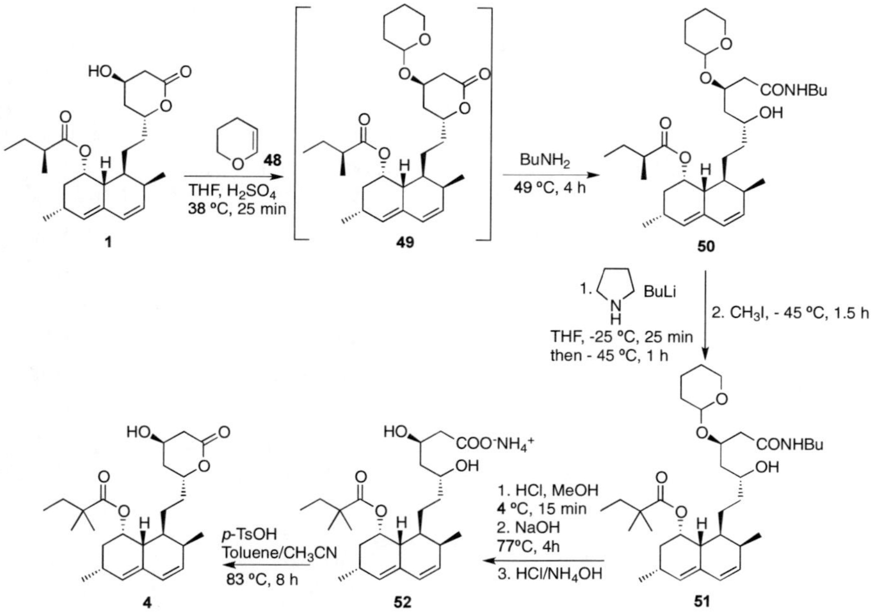

Scheme 14. Synthesis of simvastatin using 3,4-dihydro-2*H*-pyrane as protecting group.

The preparation of stable labeled simvastatin was required for pharmacological studies concerning identification and quantification of the drug and its metabolites or tissue distribution of these compounds in experimental animals. Prakash and Ellsworth described the synthesis of simvastatin labeled with ^{14}C in 1998. [21] Using a one-step methylation and [^{14}C]-methyl iodide the unprotected form of open chain lovastatin **53** was transformed into labeled simvastatin **54** in 23% radiochemical yield, which was further transformed into the labeled acid form **55**, Scheme 15.

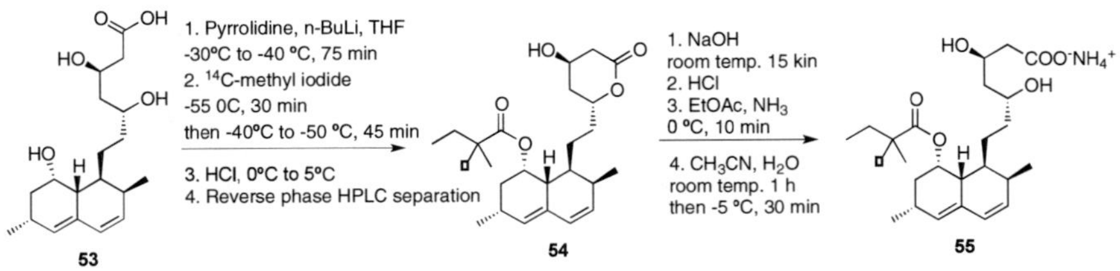

Scheme 15. Preparation of [^{14}C]simvastatin.

In order to perform the identification and quantification of simvastatin metabolites by liquid chromatography-mass spectrometry (LC-MS), it was necessary to develop methods for the synthesis of derivatives with molecular masses different from that of simvastatin. [22] The preparation of deuterium labeled simvastatin was obtained through esterification of monosilylated diol **7** with deuterium labeled 2,2-dimethylbutanoyl chloride **60**. The preparation of the labeled acyl derivative from [$^{2}H_6$]acetone **56** involved four steps, alkylation with magnesium bromide followed by chlorination and treatment with magnesium and CO_2 to afford [$^{2}H_6$]2,2-dimethylbutanoic acid **59** in 33.9% yield, which after treatment with oxalyl chloride produced [$^{2}H_6$]2,2-dimethylbutyryl chloride **60** in 95% yield, Scheme 16.

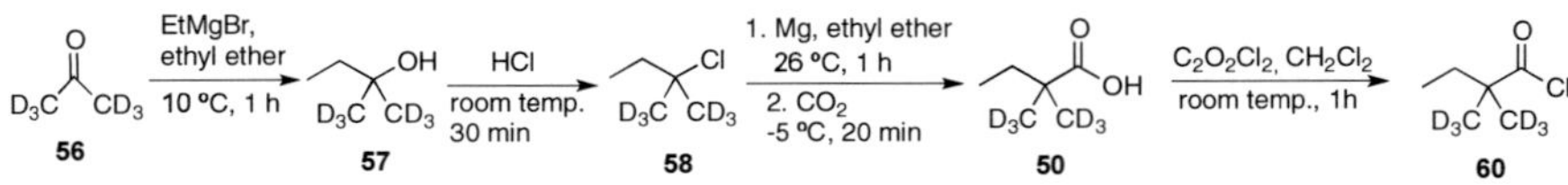

Scheme 16. Synthesis of [$^{2}H_6$]2,2-dimethylbutyryl chloride.

From the reaction of [$^{2}H_6$]2,2-dimethylbutyryl chloride **60** with the monosilylated diol **7** in pyridine and DMAP at 90 °C during 8 h protected and labeled simvastatin derivative **61** was obtained in 68.1 % yield. Deprotection was achieved using the established method with 70.5% yield, Scheme 17.

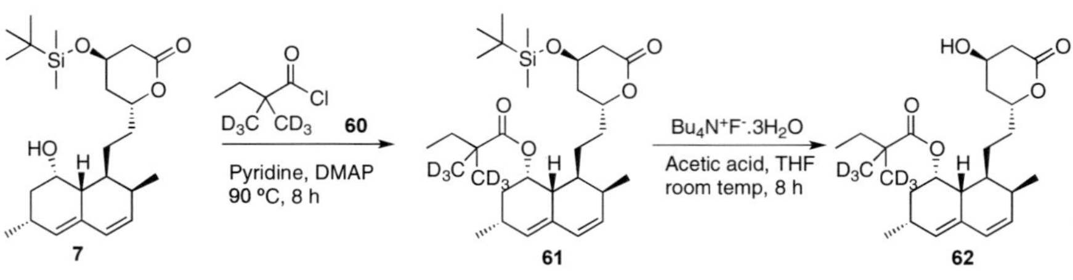

Scheme 17. Synthesis of [$^{2}H_6$]simvastatin.

Synthesis of Simvastatin Using a Biocatalyst

Simvastatin, as the second-largest selling statin in the world, bringing in millions of prescriptions and billions in sales per year, has to be produced in thousands of tons per year. Looking for improving manufacturing sustainability, Yi Tang and coworkers conceived a synthesis of simvastatin that used an engineered enzyme and a practical, low-cost feedstock. He partnered with Codexis Inc. — a developer of industrial enzymes that enables the cost-advantage production of biofuels, bio-based chemicals and pharmaceutical intermediates — to optimize both the enzyme and the chemical process for commercial use. For the development of the sustainable process for the production of simvastatin, they were presented the Presidential Green Chemistry Challenge award in 2012 in the Greener Synthetic Pathways Category, established to recognize and promote innovative chemical technologies that prevent pollution and have broad applicability in industry. It is sponsored by the EPA Office of Chemical Safety and Pollution Prevention, in partnership with the ACS Green Chemistry Institute and other members of the chemical community.

This novel method takes advantage of knowledge on the biosynthesis of lovastatin. The yeast, *saccharomyces cerevisiae*, is engineered to be able to heterologously express functional fungal polyketide synthases (PKSs). Expressing all the necessary lovastatin genes in yeast and feeding the appropriate organic side chain donor, simvastatin was directly produced. In 2006, Tang et al. cloned lovD gene from *Aspergillus terreus*, and overexpressed this enzyme in *E. coli*. [23] In this way, they were able to characterize this acyltransferase that selectively transfers the α-methylbutyryl group to the C8 hydroxyl group of menacolin J, to yield lovastatin. The authors showed that LovD has broad substrate specificity towards the acyl group. Most notably, LovD was able to catalyze the direct acylation of monacolin J (**53**) by acyl-CoA thioesters or membrane permeable thioesters acyl donors like *N*-acetylcysteamine thioesters. This work showed the feasibility of using LovD as a biocatalyst for a single-step synthesis of simvastatin using α-dimethylbutyryl-*S*-methylthioglycolate as a substrate. The authors improved the process making it faster and cheaper by deleting gene bioH from *E. coli*, generating strain YT2. In this way, 15 mM menacolin J and 25 mM 2,2-dimethylbutyrate-*S*-methyl mercaptopropionate (**63**) were transformed in to 15 mM simvastatin in 12 h. [24] A further improvement of the process consisted in an increase in the concentration of soluble LovD expressed in E. coli, Scheme 18. [25]

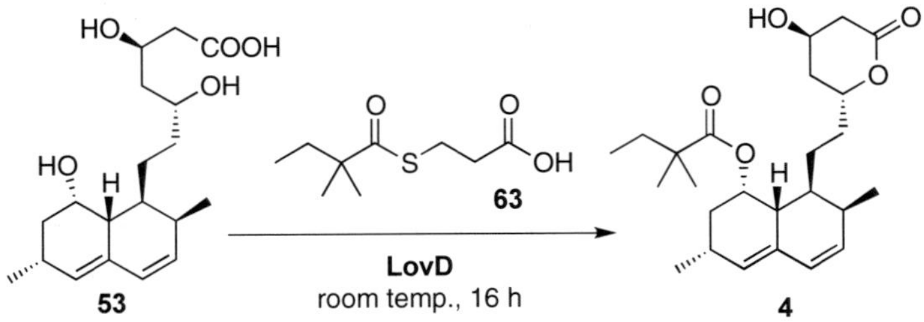

Scheme 18. Acylation using 2,2-dimethylbutyrate-*S*-methyl mercaptopropionate and biocatalyst LovD.

Van den Berg and coworkers used a different approach, engineering Aspergillus terreus so that it could directly produce simvastatin instead of lovastatin by fermentation. The authors propose inactivation of lovF gene, to prevent internal accumulation of 2- methylbutyrate together with the engineering of the Aspergillus terreus strain so that it will synthesize 2,2-dimethylbutyrate. [26]

The resulting process, which has already produced more than 10 metric tons of simvastatin, uses a catalyst produced efficiently from renewable feedstocks, reduces the use of toxic and hazardous substances such as *tert*-butyldimethylsilane chloride, methyl iodide or *n*-butyl lithium, reduces solvent waste due to the aqueous nature of the reaction conditions, improves energy efficiency as the reaction is run at ambient temperature and near atmospheric pressure; the only by-product (methyl 3-mercaptopropionic acid) can be recycled, is cost-effective, and meets the needs of millions of consumers. At present, the process is being used in Europe and India, and it may lead to an annual production of several hundreds of tons of simvastatin.

Conclusion

In the last twenty-four years several processes for the synthesis of simvastatin from lovastatin have been developed. The different semi-synthetic methods used over the years in the production of this compound can be divided into two large groups, the methylation and acylation methods and were used for the production of tons of simvastatin. The development of biocatalysts for the acylation reaction makes the production of simvastatin a more sustainable process, meeting current environmental concerns.

References

[1] Albers-Schonberg, G.; Joshua, H.; Lopez, M. B. US 4,294,846, *Merck & Co., Inc.*)1980.

[2] Albers-Schonberg, G.; Joshua, H.; Lopez, M. B. US 4,420,491, (*Merck & Co., Inc.*)1983.

[3] Wikrg, K. B.; Laidig, K. E. Acidity of (Z)- and (E)-methyl acetates: relationship to Meldrum's acid, *J. Am. Chem. Soc.* 1988, 110: 1872-1874.

[4] Sleteinger, M.; Verhoeven, T. R.; Volante, R. P. US4582915, (*Merck & Co., Inc.*), 1986.

[5] Hoffman, W. F.; Smith, R. L.; Willard, A. K. US 4,444,784, *(Merck & Co., Inc.)* 1984.

[6] Willard, A. K.; Smith, R. L. Incorporation of 2(*S*)-methylbutanoic acid-1-^{14}C into the structure of mevinolin, *J. Labell. Comp. Radiopharm.* 1982, 19: 337-344.

[7] Hoffman, W.F.; Alberts, A. W.; Anderson, P.S.; Smith, R.L.; Chen, J.S.; Willard, A.K.; 3-Hydroxy-3-methylglutaryl-coenzyme A reductase inhibitors. 4. Side chain ester derivatives of Mevinolin. *J. Med. Chem.* 1986, 29: 849-852.

[8] Zlicar, M. WO2000032585 (Lek Tovarna Farmacevtskih) 2000.

[9] a) Askin, D.; Verhoeven, T. R.; Liu, T. M. –H.; Shinkai, I. Synthesis of synvinolin: Extremely high conversion alkylation of an ester enolate, J. Org. Chem. 1991, 56: 4929-4932; b) Verhoeven, T. R.; Askin, D. US4820850 (*Merck & Co., Inc.),* 1989.

[10] Thaper, R. K.; Misra, S.; Kumar, Y.; Kumar, S. M. D.; Khanna, J. M.; A cost-efficient synthesis of simvastatin via high-conversion methylation of an alkoxide ester enolate, *Org. Process Res. Dev.* 1999, 3: 476-479.

[11] Dabora, R. L.; Tewalt, G. L. US005159104 (Merck & Co., Inc.) 1992

[12] Doucette, G.; Tam, T.F.; Tao, Y.; Karimian, K.; Li, Y. WO1999065892 (*Apotex Inc.)* 1999.

[13] Kubela, R.; Radhakrishnan, J. US005393893 (*Apotex, Inc.)* 1995.

[14] Horne, S. E.; Murthy, K. S. K.; Weeratunga, G.; Young, S. WO1998012188 (*Brantford Chem. Inc.)* 1998

[15] Dabak, K.; Adiyaman, M.; A new method for the synthesis of antihypercholesterolemic agent simvastatin. *Helv. Chim. Acta* 2003, 86: 673-677.

[16] a) Sambasivan, G.; Sridharan, M.; Acharya, P.; Mathew, J. (Biocon India Limited) US6573392, 2003; b) Sambasivan, G.; Sridharan, M.; Acharya, P.; Mathew, J. (*Biocon India Limited*) US6603022, 2003.

[17] Kim, J. W.; Bae, H.; Lee, K.H.; Choi, K.D. (*Cheil Jedang Corp.*); WO 2001072734, 2001.

[18] Taoka, N.; Inoue, K. US6331641 (*Kaneka Corporation*), 2001

[19] Zupačnič, S.; Stimac, A.; Gnidovec, J. US 6252091, KRKA, (Tovarna Zdravil, D.D.) 2001.

[20] Singamsetty, R. K.; Vujjini, S. K.; Manne, N. Naga, B. R. M. V.; Himabindu, V.; Battacharya, A.; Ghanta, M. R.; Bandichhor, R. New synthesis of simvastatin. *Synthetic Commun.* 2008: 38, 4452-4459.

[21] Prakash, S. R.; Ellsworth R. L. Carbon-14 methylation of the 2-methylbutyryl side chain of mevinolin and its analogs, *J. Labelled Comp. Radiopharm.* 1998, 25: 815-825.

[22] Tian, L.; Tao, J.; Chen, L. Synthesis of deuterium-labeled simvastatin, *J. Labell. Comp. Radiopharm.* 2011, 54: 625-628.

[23] Xie, X.; Watanabe, K.; Wojcicki, W. A.; Wang, C. C. C.; Tang, Y. Biosynthesis of Lovastatin analogs with a broadly specific acyltransferase, *Chem. Biol.* 2006, 13: 1161-1169.

[24] Xie X.; Tang, Y., Efficient synthesis of simvastatin using whole-cell biocatalysis. *Appl Environ Microbiol,* 2007, 73: 2054–2060.

[25] Xie, X.; Meehan, M. J.; Xu, W.; Dorrestein, P. C.; Tang, Y. Acyltransferase-mediated polyketide release from a fungal megasynthase. *J. Am. Chem. Soc.* 2009, 131: 8388-8389.

[26] Van den Berg, M. A.; Hans, M.; Streekstra, H. WO 2007147801A1, (Dsm Ip Assets Bv, Van Den Marco Alexander Berg, Marcus Hans, Hugo Streekstra) 2007.

In: Simvastatin Delivery
Editors: Alberto A. C. C. Pais et al.
ISBN: 978-1-63482-148-3

Chapter 2

The Pharmacology of Simvastatin: From the Mechanism of Action to New Therapeutic Applications

Ana Fortuna[1,2], Gilberto Alves[2,3] and Amílcar Falcão[1,2]***

[1] Laboratory of Pharmacology, Faculty of Pharmacy, University of Coimbra, Pólo das Ciências da Saúde, Azinhaga de Santa Comba, Coimbra, Portugal
[2] CNC – Centre for Neuroscience and Cell Biology, University of Coimbra, Coimbra, Portugal
[3] CICS-UBI – Health Sciences Research Centre, University of Beira Interior, Covilhã, Portugal

Abstract

Simvastatin is a lipid lowering agent with an excellent safety profile, which is widely used in the clinical practice for treatment of dyslipidemia and prevention of cardiovascular diseases. Recently, other

* Laboratory of Pharmacology, Faculty of Pharmacy, University of Coimbra, Pólo das Ciências da Saúde, Azinhaga de Santa Comba, 3000-548 Coimbra, Portugal; Email: acfalcao@ff.uc.pt.

pharmacological actions have been ascribed to simvastatin including antioxidant, immunomodulatory, anticoagulant, anti-inflammatory, and neuroprotective properties. These pleiotropic effects result from the inhibition of the synthesis of important isoprenoid intermediates besides cholesterol and they are currently making simvastatin an appealing drug candidate for patients with neurological diseases, such as Alzheimer's disease, dementia, Parkinson's disease and multiple sclerosis, as well as in bone diseases and tumor therapy.

In the present chapter, the pharmacodynamic, pharmacokinetic and safety properties of simvastatin will be revised and compared with those of other statins as well as the cellular mechanisms underlying the hypolipidemic and pleiotropic activities. Finally, (non-)clinical evidence regarding the new clinical applications of simvastatin will be also revised and discussed.

Keywords: Simvastatin; HMG-CoA reductase inhibitors; pharmacokinetics; hypolipidemic effect; pleiotropic effects

Abbreviations

Aß	Alzheimer's amyloid peptide
AMPK	AMP-protein kinase
AUC	area under the plasma concentration-time curve
BBB	blood-brain barrier
BMP	bone morphogenetic protein
BMP-2	morphogenetic protein type 2
CNS	central nervous system
CYP	cytochrome P450
eNOS	endothelial nitric oxide synthase
EPC	endothelial progenitor cells
FPP	farnesyl pyrophosphate
GELs	gadolinium-enhancing lesions
GGPP	geranylgeranyl pyrophosphate
GTP	guanosine triphosphate
HDL-C	high-density lipoprotein cholesterol
HIV	human immunodeficiency virus
HMG-CoA	3-hydroxy-3-methyl-glutaryl-coenzyme A
IC50	half maximal inhibition concentration
IFN-γ	interferon gamma

iNOS	inducible or inflammatory nitric oxide synthase
LDL-C	low-density lipoprotein cholesterol
MHC	major histocompatibility complex
MMRS	relapsing-remitting multiple sclerosis
NADPH	nicotinamide dinucleotide phosphate
NF-kB	nuclear factor-kappa B
nNOS	neuronal nitric oxide synthase
NO	nitric oxide
PAI-1	plasminogen activator inhibitor 1
PI3K/Akt	phosphatidylinositol 3-kinase/protein kinase Akt
ROCK	Rho-associated kinase
ROS	reactive oxygen species
TF	tissue factor
TFPI	tissue factor pathway inhibitor
TNF-α	tumour necrosis factor alfa
tPA	tissue-type plasminogen activator
VLDL	very-low-density lipoproteins
VSMC	vascular smooth muscle cells

Introduction

Similarly to the other six statins currently marketed, simvastatin is worldwide used for the management of cardiovascular risk and for the prevention of coronary heart diseases and atherosclerotic disorders related to the hypercholesterolemia. As a competitive inhibitor of the enzyme 3-hydroxy-3-methyl-glutaryl-coenzyme A (HMG-CoA) reductase, which catalyses the rate-limiting step in cholesterol biosynthesis, simvastatin is a cholesterol-lowering agent with current proven efficacy and safety profiles. Approved since 1988, simvastatin has demonstrated to reduce the risks of vascular death, non-fatal myocardial infarction and the need for arterial revascularization in large randomized trials [1,2]. In the clinical trials, it became clear that the extent of risk reduction was directly proportional to the degree to which the low-density lipoprotein cholesterol (LDL-C) was lowered.

Although the commonly known pharmacological activity of simvastatin relies on its potent inhibition effects on the endogenous mevalonate pathway, preventing the biosynthesis of cholesterol (Figure 1), a multifaceted action on different physiological and pathological conditions has been recently evidenced. Indeed, statins have shown to affect several tissue functions and modulate specific signal transduction pathways through cholesterol-independent mechanisms, involving other products of the mevalonate pathway, namely the non-steroid isoprenoid metabolites such as the farnesyl pyrophosphate (FPP) and the geranylgeranyl pyrophosphate (GGPP) (Figure 1). These cholesterol-independent effects mediated by statins are known as pleiotropic effects and include, among others, the anti-inflammatory, immunomodulatory, vasculoprotective, anti-platelet and antioxidant effects which may improve the endothelial function, inhibit vascular inflammation and oxidation and stabilize atherosclerotic plaques [3]. Thus, in addition to their potent anti-atherosclerotic and cardio-protective actions, emerging evidence is revealing that those beneficial properties have potential therapeutic implications in bone diseases, tumours and neurological pathological conditions including dementia, Alzheimer's disease, Parkinson's disease and multiple sclerosis.

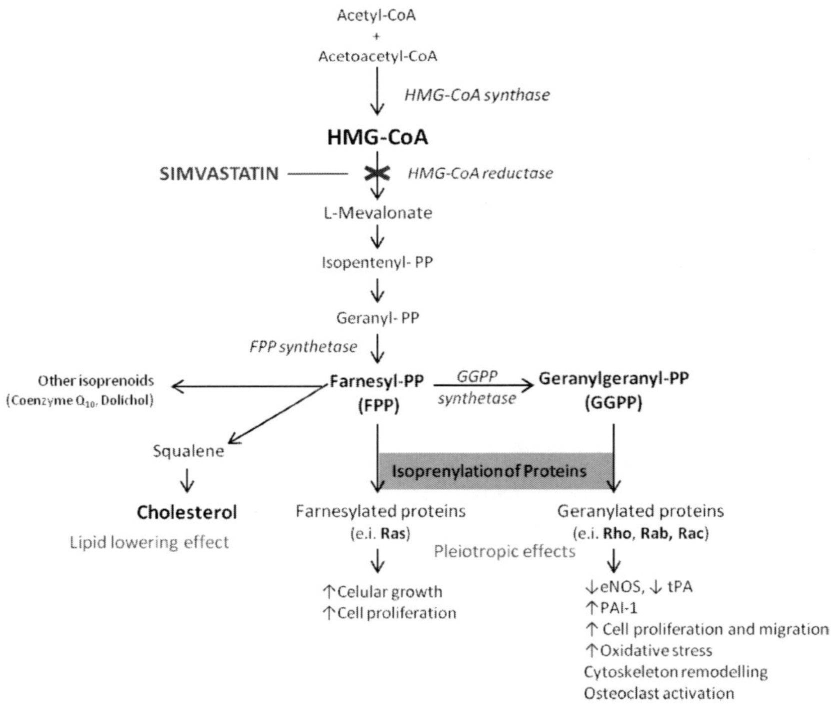

Figure 1. The interaction between the HMG-CoA reductase and simvastatin, in the mammalian mevalonate pathway. (eNOS, endothelial nitric oxide synthase; HMG-CoA, 3-hydroxy-3-methylglutaryl-coenzyme A; PAI-1, plasminogen activator inhibitor 1; PP, pyrophosphate; tPA, tissue-type plasminogen activator).

In the present chapter, the pharmacodynamic, pharmacokinetic and safety properties of simvastatin will be revised as well as the cellular mechanisms underlying its hypolipidemic and pleiotropic activities. Moreover, compelling non-clinical and clinical studies particularly regarding new clinical applications of simvastatin will be also revised and discussed. Although simvastatin acts through the same mechanism of action of the other statins and shares many features with them, it also exhibits distinct pharmacological attributes that may differentiate its potency, effectiveness and clinical utility. Therefore, while describing the pharmacology of simvastatin throughout this chapter, the respective characteristics will be compared with those of the remaining HMG-CoA reductase inhibitors.

Pharmacological Properties and Chemical Structure of Simvastatin

Due to its powerful lipid-lowering activity that can decrease LDL-C levels by up to 50%, simvastatin, marketed under several trade names such as Zocor®, Simlup®, Simcard® and Simvacor®, is commonly prescribed to control hypercholesterolemia. Usually, patients start the treatment at the dose of 20 mg per day, but it commonly varies from 10 to 80 mg, which is the highest approved dosage for simvastatin. However, doses of 80 mg and higher (up to 160 mg) have been found to be too toxic while giving only minimal benefits regarding lipid-lowering therapy [4].

The therapeutic target organ of all the statins, including simvastatin, is the liver, since it is the major site of endogenous cholesterol biosynthesis. The synthesis of cholesterol in the body is initiated through a biochemical reaction involving one molecule of acetyl-coenzyme A and one molecule of acetoacetyl-coenzyme A (Figure 1), but the process involves 28 steps. Statins block the second step of conversion of HMG-CoA into mevalonate by inhibiting the enzyme HMG-CoA reductase that catalyses this reaction (Figure 1). The inhibition of the endogenous de novo synthesis of cholesterol is important since the most circulating cholesterol comes from the internal manufacture rather than from diet [5]. This reduction in the intracellular cholesterol concentration yields a homeostatic increase in LDL-receptors cycling on the hepatocyte cell surface. These receptors recognize and bind to apolipoproteins B and E on the surface of circulating very-low-density lipoproteins (VLDL) and low-density lipoproteins (LDL), increasing the extraction of LDL-C from the blood into the cell and, consequently, decreasing its circulating concentrations [6]. In addition, simvastatin produces a modest increase on the concentrations of the high-density lipoprotein cholesterol (HDL-C). In fact, it is one of the statins with higher potency at this level (Table 1). Two mechanisms seem to be involved in this increment. The first one is related to the enhancement of apolipoprotein A production. Since this apolipoprotein is the major one in HDL, the respective increment induces the production of nascent HDL and consequently increases HDL-C. The second potential mechanism for increasing HDL-C bases on reducing the transference of cholesterol esters from HDL to VLDL and LDL particles via inhibition of cholesteryl ester transfer protein. Simvastatin also demonstrated to have beneficial effects on decreasing the triglyceride concentrations in serum (Table 1). All together, these pharmacological activities make simvastatin clinically useful to reduce the elevated total-cholesterol, LDL-C and triglycerides and increase HDL-C in patients with primary hyperlipidemia and mixed dyslipidemia which is characterized by elevated LDL-C and triglyceride levels [12].

While these effects on plasma cholesterol are well documented and have been recently reviewed, there exists emerging evidence that the inhibition of the mevalonate pathway may provide positive pleiotropic effects that are independent of cholesterol. Indeed, concomitantly with the reduction of cholesterol synthesis, the blockade of HMG-CoA reductase also decreases the synthesis of non-sterol isoprenoids (Figure 1). As these compounds are the major donors of prenyl groups for protein prenylation activation, their reduction in synthesis underlies many of the pleiotropic effects of simvastatin and the remaining statins in general. Due to its complexity and wide range of consequences, this point will be detailed in section 5 of the present chapter.

Chemically, simvastatin is the [(1S,3R,7S,8S,8aR)-8-[2-[(2R,4R)-4-hydroxy -6 –oxooxan -2- yl] ethyl] -3,7-dimethyl -1, 2, 3, 7, 8, 8a-hexa-hydronaphthalen -1-yl] 2,2-dimethylbutanoate (Figure 2). Administered as the inactive lactone prodrug, simvastatin is rapidly hydrolyzed in the liver and non-hepatic tissues to its active ß-hydroxyacid form which inhibits the HMG-CoA reductase (Figure 2). Its structure can be broadly divided into two parts: the pharmacophore, which is a dihydroxyheptanoic acid segment with two chiral carbon atoms; and, covalently linked to the pharmacophore, is a moiety composed of a partially reduced naphthalene hydrophobic ring attached to the 2,2-methylbutyrate ester. Common to all statins, the pharmacophore is structurally analogue to the target enzyme substrate (HMG-CoA), allowing the drug to inhibit the HMG-CoA reductase in a competitive, dose-dependent and reversible manner (Figure 2). Moreover, although the stereochemistry of simvastatin on its pharmacophore is dictated by the stereoselectivity of the enzyme, the partially reduced naphthalene ring is also involved in the formation of the simvastatin-enzyme complex since it keeps the drug close to the enzyme, precluding the possibility of simvastatin displacement by the endogenous substrate. Crystallographic studies on the simvastatin-HMG-CoA reductase complex demonstrated that simvastatin binds to the enzyme through van der Waals interactions [13]. On the other hand, the groups on the rings determine the solubility properties of the drugs and, therefore, their pharmacokinetic profiles and tissue-selectivity. The group 2,2-methylbutirate ester of simvastatin confers itself a high lipophilicity and a substantial increment in the potency of the drug.

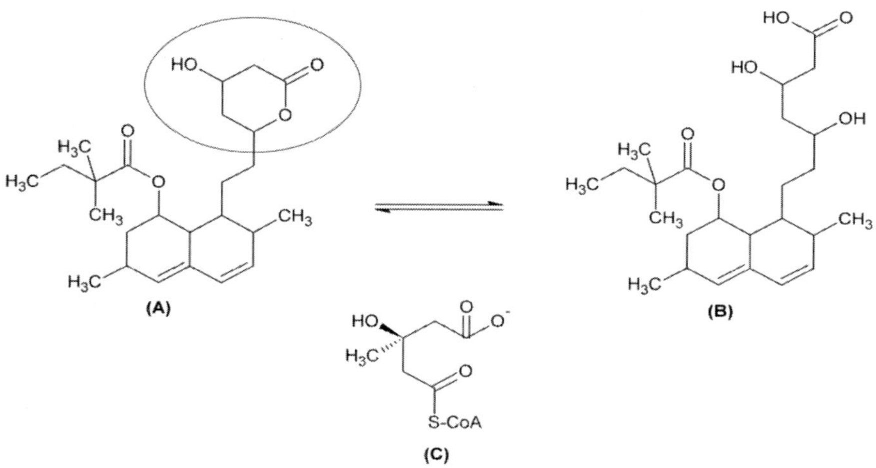

Figure 2. Chemical structure of simvastatin (A) and its corresponding active ß-hydroxyacid form (B) which inhibits the HMG-CoA (C) reductase. HMG-CoA-like pharmacophore that is conserved in all statins is included in the cycle.

At this point, it is important to highlight that although all the statins share the same pharmacophore group, different groups may constitute their moieties, influencing their mode of binding to the enzyme and consequently their potency and pharmacokinetics. Indeed, the subtle differences that exist in the number and types of bonds explain the different potency of statins to lower LDL-C in a way that a larger degree of binding to the enzyme translates into a higher potency (Table 1). Simvastatin is a natural lipid-lowering agent derived from a fermentation product of *Aspergillus terreus*. It is a natural fungal metabolite, as well as lovastatin and pravastatin, and it is more potent as inhibitor of HMG-CoA reductase than pravastatin, exhibiting a lower half maximal inhibition concentration (IC_{50}) in vitro and in vivo (Table 1). The discovery of the intrinsic ability of natural statins to inhibit the enzyme HMG-CoA reductase prompted the development of the synthetic statins as atorvastatin, fluvastatin, rosuvastatin and cerivastatin (which was withdrawn from the market due to its severe adverse effects). The structural design of these statins has been modelled to achieve different functionalities tightly related to each particular component of the molecule. The functional difference between synthetic and natural statins resides on their affinity to the target enzyme and their lipophilicity. As summarized in Table 1, the potency of simvastatin is quite lower when compared to those of the synthetic statins. For instance the pyrrole and pyrimidine rings present on atorvastatin and rosuvastatin molecules, respectively, render them additional hydrogen binding interactions that increase their affinity to the HMG-CoA reductase when compared to simvastatin. Moreover, the methane sulfonamide group of rosuvastatin allows an additional polar interaction with the enzyme, making it the most potent HMG-CoA reductase inhibitor [14,15].

Table 1. Comparative chemical structure, lipophilicity and effectiveness on statin drugs [7-11]

				Effect on various lipid fractions (%)		
Statin	**Ring**	**Lipophilicity** (log P)	**IC_{50}**[a]	**↓ LDL-C**	**↑ HDL-C**	**↓ Triglyceride**
Atorvastatin	Pyrrole	1.11	15.2	50	6	29
Cerivastatin*	Pyridine	1.69	13.1	28	10	13
Fluvastatin	Indole	1.27	17.9	24	8	10
Lovastatin	Naphthalene	1.70	2.7-11.1	34	9	16
Pitavastatin	Quinoline	1.49	6.8	48	-	23
Pravastatin	Naphthalene	-0.84	55.1	34	12	24
Rosuvastatin	Pyrimidine	-0.33	12.0	63	10	28
Simvastatin	**Naphthalene**	**1.60**	**18.1**	**41**	**12**	**18**

HDL-C, high-density lipoprotein cholesterol; IC_{50}, half maximal inhibitory concentration; LDL-C, low-density lipoprotein cholesterol; log P, *n*-octanol/water partition coefficient of the active hydroxy forms of statins;
* withdrawn from the market; ↓- reduction; ↑ - increase;
[a] Results in relation to HMG-CoA reductase inhibition (nM).

Pharmacokinetics and Tissue-Selectivity

Simvastatin is administered orally as a lactone prodrug, rapidly and moderately absorbed in the intestine. It reaches the peak plasma concentration within 1.3-2.4 h post-dosing and exhibits a percentage of absorption between 65 and 85% (Table 2) [9,16,17]. This absorption range, in opposition to those of several statins, is not affected by food. Instead, clinical studies performed in patients with hypercholesterolemia revealed that the absorption of simvastatin depends on the age and sex of the individuals, with plasma concentrations enhanced in elderly persons (70-78 years old) and women [18]. Although these influences contribute to a slightly wide absorption range, they do not imply modifications on the dosage regimens.

Interestingly, the systemic bioavailability stands out as the lowest one among all the statins (< 5%), indicating that simvastatin suffers an extensive first-pass extraction in the liver (Table 2). This results from two main characteristics of the drug. Firstly, as a prodrug, it must be rapidly biotransformed to the main active metabolites which include the ß-hydroxyacid and its 6'-hydroxy, 6'-hydroxymethyl and 6'-exomethylene derivatives [19]. Secondly, simvastatin is very lipophilic and, therefore, it is passively diffused into the hepatocytes where it can be metabolized or it can prosecute its inhibitory activity on HMG-CoA reductase. The low systemic absorption is not a disadvantage in this case. In fact, because the liver is the target organ of statins, an efficient first-pass hepatic uptake is, generally, more important and desirable than high systemic bioavailability. For instance, cerivastatin, which was removed from the market due to its unacceptable frequency of severe muscle toxicity, exhibited a 60% systemic bioavailability (Table 2). Nevertheless, the lipophilicity of simvastatin also confers it a high ability to penetrate cells of extrahepatic tissues even though the drug is extensively bound to plasma proteins (Table 2). Thus, while lipophilicity results in an efficient hepatic shunting, it may also contribute for the development of undesirable systemic adverse effects and beneficial pleiotropic effects. In opposition to simvastatin, hydrophilic statins are much more hepatoselective because they are excluded from the peripheral tissues; for instance the lack of influence of pravastatin on smooth muscle cell proliferation has been attributed to its low penetration on the tissue [11]. Moreover, an in vivo study performed in rats revealed that rosuvastatin and pravastatin (hydrophilic statins as observed by their *n*-octanol/water partition coefficient depicted in Table 1) exhibited liver selective uptake after intravenous administration, while simvastatin exhibited higher uptake rates in liver and in other tissues, namely adrenals and spleen [20]. Importantly, another study in the same animal model indicated that, when radiolabeled simvastatin was administered, radioactivity was detected in the brain [12]. The lipophilicity of simvastatin, as well as that of lovastatin, seems to be the main determinant for their higher ability to permeate the blood-brain barrier (BBB) in relation to the remaining statins [17]. Moreover, the negative charge of the statin (for example fluvastatin) may also hamper its passage into the brain since it would be repelled by the anionic microdomains in the plasma membrane of BBB endothelial cells [21]. This variation of statin properties can explain why simvastatin shows some beneficial effects on the central nervous system (CNS) diseases in opposition to other statins. This point will be outlined in the last section of this chapter.

In the liver, simvastatin lactone is chemically or enzymatically hydrolysed to its open acid form by esterases or paraoxonases. In addition, it rapidly undergoes oxidation through the microsomal cytochrome P450 (CYP), specifically by the isoenzyme 3A4 (CYP3A4) [7,22]. This fact is not surprising considering that lipophilic drugs are known to be very susceptible to oxidative metabolism by CYP. Indeed, consulting Table 2, it becomes evident that CYP metabolizes almost all the statins in spite of the different isoenzymes that may be involved; however, for the hydrophilic pravastatin, rosuvastatin and pitavastatin, the contribution of CYP isoenzymes is negligible.

The half-life elimination time of simvastatin is only 1.9-3.0 h (Table 2) and, consequently, it must be administered in the evening when the rate of endogenous cholesterol synthesis is higher. Although the predominant route of elimination of simvastatin is via the bile after hepatic metabolism into the faeces (60%), approximately 13% of the dose is also excreted in urine (Table 2). This makes simvastatin contraindicated in patients with hepatic dysfunction, since its plasma levels are enhanced and, consequently, there is an increased risk for inducing lateral effects, namely myopathy. In opposition, because simvastatin does not undergo significant renal excretion, modification of dosage should not be necessary in patients with mild to moderate renal impairment; however, caution must be exercised when the drug is administered to patients with severe renal impairment, who should be closely monitored [12].

Table 2. Comparative pharmacokinetic characteristics of statin drugs [9,16,17]

	Atorvastatin	Cerivastatin*	Fluvastatin	Lovastatin	Pitavastatin	Pravastatin	Rosuvastatin	Simvastatin
Absorption (%)	30	> 98	98	31	80	37	50	65-85
t_{max} (h)	2.4-4.0	2.5-3.0	0.5-1.5	2.8	0.5-0.8	0.9-1.6	3	1.3-2.4
F (%)	12	60	10-35	< 5	>60	17	20	< 5
Food effect on *F*	↓ 13%	No	↓15-25%	↑ 50%	No	↓ 30%	No	No
Protein binding (%)	> 98	> 99.5	> 98	96-98.5	96	43-54	88	> 95
BBB Permeable	Controversial	Controversial	No	Yes	NF	Limited	Limited	Yes
CYP isoenzyme	CYP3A4	CYP3A4 CYP2C8	CYP2C9	CYP3A4	CYP2C9 minimally	CYP3A4 minimally	CYP2C9 minimally	CYP3A4
Active metabolites	Yes	Yes	Yes	Yes	No	Yes	No	Yes
Renal excretion (%)	2	24	6	30	< 2	60	10	13
$t_{1/2}$ (h)	11-30	2.0-3.0	0.5-2.3	2.5-3.0	11	0.8-3.0	20	1.9-3.0

BBB, blood-brain barrier; CYP, cytochrome P450; *F*, systemic bioavailability; NF, not found; t_{max} , time to reach the peak plasma concentration; $t_{1/2}$, half-life elimination time;
*withdrawn from the market; ↓- reduction; ↑ - increase.

Safety of Simvastatin

Simvastatin is well tolerated; indeed, although its only well-documented and consistent adverse effects are serious, they are rare at standard doses [7]. They include muscle toxicity, namely myopathy which may progress to rhabdomyolysis, and hepatotoxicity characterized by an increase of hepatic enzymes.

Myopathy is defined as any muscle symptom (pain, tenderness or weakness) accompanied by a creatine kinase concentration greater than ten times the upper limit considered normal. It may progress to rhabdomyolysis that involves muscle breakdown and myoglobin release to systemic circulation, causing a brown discoloration of urine and risk of renal failure. The hepatotoxicity of simvastatin occurred as a persistent increase in serum transaminases in approximately 1% of patients who received simvastatin in clinical studies. Therefore, although interruption of the drug treatment slowly reduces the transaminases levels to pre-treatment levels, it is recommended to perform liver function tests before and during the treatment [23].

Importantly, these adverse effects are generally due to excessive simvastatin dosing or drug-drug interactions that inhibit simvastatin metabolism. Indeed, in one clinical trial (n = 4497), simvastatin was administered to patients with acute coronary syndrome at the dose of 40 mg for one month, increasing to 80 mg daily or placebo for 4 months; thereafter simvastatin was administered at 20 mg daily for at least 2 years. The study revealed an enhanced myopathy risk with simvastatin 80 mg daily, reporting nine cases of myopathy against only one in the group that received placebo [24]. This is supported by the product information for simvastatin which gives an estimated incidence of myopathy with 80 mg daily as 0.53% and 0.08% at the dose of 40 mg daily.

On the other hand, as aforementioned in the previous section, simvastatin is mainly metabolized by CYP3A4, which is responsible for the metabolism of the majority of drugs in humans. Thus, the co-administration of CYP3A4 inhibitors with simvastatin leads to an increase of statin plasma levels, bioavailability and, consequently, the risk of related adverse events. A similar interaction may occur between simvastatin and other substrates of CYP3A4 by competing for the same metabolic mechanism. It is worthy to note that simvastatin is regarded, together with lovastatin, as the statin with the highest potential for clinically relevant interactions [25]. The remaining statins may be metabolized by CYP3A4 but the effect of CYP3A4 inhibitors on their plasma levels may not be so evident because other metabolic enzymes may also be involved and compensate the inhibition of CYP3A4. Among the CYP3A4 inhibitors, are the antifungal agents (itraconazole and ketoconazole), cyclosporine, macrolide antibiotics (erythromycin and clarithromycin), human immunodeficiency virus (HIV) protease inhibitors and grapefruit juice. In the particular case of simvastatin, its co-administration with itraconazole results in a 19-fold increase of the area under the plasma concentration-time curve (AUC), causing rhabdomyolysis [26,27]. Similar effects have been reported when simvastatin is associated to erythromycin and clarithromycin [22], the bacteriostatic antibiotic fusidic acid [28] and the HIV protease inhibitor nelfinavir which considerably increased the simvastatin plasma concentration [29]. These combinations are therefore contraindicated. However if short-term treatment with strong CYP3A4 inhibitors is unavoidable, therapy with simvastatin must be suspended during the course of the treatment. The effect of calcium channel antagonists (verapamil and diltiazem), which also inhibit CYP3A4, on the pharmacokinetics of simvastatin has also been reported, showing an increase of simvastatin plasma levels and the risks of associated rhabdomyolysis and hepatitis [25,30]. Importantly, Hickmott et al. [31] outlined the reduced clearance of simvastatin (around 60%) and R-warfarin (between 10 and 20%) after their co-administration, since both drugs are substrate of CYP3A4. Simvastatin-drug interactions associated with CYP3A4 inducers have also been described. For example, when co-administered with carbamazepine, the plasma AUC of simvastatin and its active metabolite were reduced as well as their cholesterol-lowering effects [32,33].

Caution is also recommended when prescribing fibrates with simvastatin, as those agents can cause myopathy when admnistered alone and the risk is increased when they are co-administered. Moreover cases of myopathy, including rhabdomyolysis, have been reported with simvastatin co-administered with colchicine, and therefore the benefits of the combined use of simvastatin with that drug should be carefully weighed against the potential risks of the combination [12].

Pleiotropic Effects of Simvastatin

Recent studies are demonstrating that the overall benefits observed with the statins treatment are larger than those that would be expected considering only alterations in lipid levels. The most relevant cholesterol-independent or pleiotropic effects of simvastatin will be particularly described throughout this section and include the increase of nitric oxide (NO) availability, the improvement of endothelial function, the reduction of platelet activation and pro-coagulation cascade, the increase of fibrinolysis and the anti-coagulation cascade, stabilization of atherosclerotic plaques as well as antioxidant, immunomodulatory and anti-inflammatory activities [34-36]. These findings led to speculate the success of simvastatin in several pathological disorders besides hypercholesterolemia, as it will be explained in section 6.

The main mechanism through which simvastatin, as well as all the statins in general, induce the pleiotropic effects consists on the depletion of other isoprenoid products besides cholesterol, because, by inhibiting mevalonate production, the synthesis of other important isoprenoid intermediates is also compromised. The seventh step of the cholesterol synthesis yields FPP which can be converted to squalene and, hence, to cholesterol or to GGPP (Figure 1). Both FPP and GGPP serve as adjuncts in the post-translational isoprenylation process of several proteins, including the γ-subunit of the heterotrimetric G proteins, the small guanosine triphosphate (GTP)-binding protein Ras and the Ras-like proteins such as Rac, Rho and Rab. Isoprenylation consists on the addition of isoprenoids to the C-terminal of these proteins and it is a critical event in their intracellular trafficking and function, enabling the proteins to translocate and anchor in the membrane, subsequently targeting them to specific subcellular locations and allowing the protein to interact with effector molecules and cytoplasmatic regulators through protein-protein and protein-lipid interactions. Particularly, the modification with FPP, named farnesylation, is necessary for an adequate function and localization of Ras family proteins while GGPP is required for the geranylgeranylation of Rho, Rab and Rac family proteins (Figure 1). FPP is also the substrate for the production of coenzyme Q_{10} and dolichol, which are an antioxidant and a radical scavenger, respectively. Rho and Rac regulate organization of cytoskeletal proteins involved in the endothelial cell barrier function, and are, in turn, involved in the inflammatory signal transduction pathways and also influence the endothelial nitric oxide synthase (eNOS) expression and consequently the availability of NO. Rho also participates in signalling pathways required for nuclear factor-kappa B (NF-kB) activation, inducing the production of cytokines and chemokines. The inhibition of the small GTP-binding proteins isoprenylation by simvastatin accumulates the inactive forms of those proteins in cytoplasm, mediating several cholesterol-independent effects in vascular wall cells, leukocytes and bone.

Regulation of the Nitric Oxide Production

NO is a key mediator of the endothelial function necessary to maintain the vascular homeostasis. Generated from L-arginine by eNOS, neuronal nitric oxide synthase (nNOS) and inducible or inflammatory nitric oxide synthase (iNOS) expressed by macrophages, NO modulates the production of reactive oxygen species (ROS), blood flow, platelet function, vascular permeability and vascular tone; moreover, it limits inflammation and coagulation and diminishes the vascular smooth muscle cell proliferation and migration [37]. Importantly, inhibition of several components of the atherogenic process has been ascribed to the endothelial NO, particularly because it promotes vascular relaxation and inhibits platelet aggregation, smooth muscle cell proliferation and endothelial leucocyte interactions [36].

Statins are known to increase the signalling molecule NO availability by increasing the eNOS expression and function, leading to the improvement of the endothelial function [38]. Simvastatin seems to increase the activity of eNOS in endothelial cells through several mechanisms. Firstly, it enhances eNOS transcripts with long poly(A) tails, increasing the stability of eNOS mRNA but not the respective gene transcription [39]. This effect appears to be mediated by inhibition of Rho GTPase and its effector, the Rho-associated kinase (ROCK) [38,40]. Secondly, the eNOS activity depends on the phosphorylation at serine/threonine residues, and simvastatin seems to induce the eNOS Ser633 phosphorylation in an AMP-protein kinase (AMPK)-mediated way, enhancing the enzymatic activity. Simvastatin also increases eNOS by activation of the Ras-mediated phosphatidylinositol 3-kinase/protein kinase Akt (PI3K/Akt) ERK1/2-RSK signalling pathways [18,37].

Up to date, simvastatin has also shown to inhibit the activity of the nicotinamide dinucleotide phosphate (NADPH)-oxidase, which is a predominant source of superoxide anion in vasculature and in the CNS [41]. The consequent suppression of superoxide anion production by simvastatin is beneficial not only because it is a scavenger of NO, limiting its availability, but also because it leads to nitrate tolerance, vasoconstriction and hypertension [36].

Apart from increasing the NO production and reducing the superoxide anion synthesis, simvastatin exhibits other antioxidant effects that ameliorate vascular function. Thus, in vascular smooth muscle cells (VSMC), simvastatin induces heme oxygenase expression, an important antioxidant defence mechanism, and increases the expression of the antioxidant enzymes, superoxide dismutase and glutathione peroxidase, in aortic rings of hypertensive rats [42].

Clearly, simvastatin favourably modulates vascular redox by improving NO availability and other antioxidant cellular defences, enhancing the elimination of reactive oxygen species.

Improvement of Endothelial Function

Improvement of the endothelial function and vasculoprotective action are well recognized as pleiotropic effects of statins. Although the reduction of LDL-C levels improves the endothelial-dependent vasodilatation suggesting that statins restore the endothelial function by lowering cholesterol plasma levels, some studies revealed that this improvement occurs before significant reduction in serum cholesterol concentration [36].

Beyond the improvement of the endothelial function promoted by the induction of eNOS and antioxidant cellular defences aforementioned, simvastatin also attenuates endothelial dysfunctions by increasing the expression of tissue-type plasminogen activator (tPA) and inhibiting the expression of endothelin-1, a potent vasoconstrictor and mitogen [36,43]. In addition, it has also been reported to affect the angiogenesis process, the biology of endothelial progenitor cells (EPCs) and the proliferation of VSMC, which, together with the remaining mechanisms, contributes to improve endothelial function.

Thus, on the long-term treatment, simvastatin seems to induce neovascularization by increasing angiogenesis and recruiting EPCs. It was firstly observed that simvastatin induced neovascularization in vitro and in the ischemic limbs of normocholesterolemic rabbits [44]. Nevertheless, it is also known that simvastatin inhibits the tumor induced angiogenesis in mice and neovascular growth through a Rho-dependent inhibition of vascular endothelial growth factor receptor, Akt and focal adhesion kinases [45]. Indeed, simvastatin effects on angiogenesis are biphasic: at low doses, it stimulates angiogenesis and inhibits the necrosis factor α-induced inflammatory angiogenesis; while, at high doses, simvastatin inhibits angiogenesis. This biphasic effect is beneficial because the angiogenic response is a protective physiological mechanism against ischemia and hence it is a therapeutic strategy for coronary artery and peripheral vascular diseases [7, 38]. On the other hand, angiogenesis may be pathological as it is involved in the pathogenesis of cancer, atherosclerosis, rheumatoid arthritis and diabetic retinopathy [7,45,46]; under these circumstances, angiogenesis inhibition by simvastatin may be therapeutically useful.

Furthermore, simvastatin promotes the mobilization of hematopoietic progenitor cells from the bone marrow, increasing EPC proliferation, survival and function probably by a mechanism that involves PI3K/Akt pathway and inhibition of apoptosis. Thereafter, the EPCs augment ischemia-induced neovascularization, accelerate re-endothelialisation and improve post-ischemic cardiac function [46-48].

Regarding the VSMCs, simvastatin has been shown to inhibit their proliferation, migration and invasion predominantly by inhibiting the prenylation of Rho and the induction of their apoptosis [7]. Importantly, simvastatin demonstrated to be able of potentiating VSMC apoptosis not only in rats but also in humans [49]. Although not fully understood, the mechanism underlying simvastatin-induction of VSMC apoptosis has been attributed to the reduced synthesis of FPP and GGPP involved in the post-translational prenylation of proteins that regulate apoptosis. In particular, simvastatin treatment has been shown to inactivate p-21 RhoA protein through inhibition of its prenylation, and subsequently down-regulates the expression of anti-apoptotic Bcl-2 protein and stimulates the expression of the tumour necrosis factor alfa (TNF-α), potentiating the apoptosis [50]. Interestingly, only the lipophilic HMG-CoA reductase inhibitors like simvastatin enhanced VSMC apoptosis, while the hydrophilic rosuvastatin and pravastatin have been reported to inhibit the apoptotic process [51]. This is extremely favourable on improving the endothelial function since VSMCs play a central role in pathogenesis of vascular diseases, including transplant arteriosclerosis, post-angioplasty restenosis and venous graft occlusion [36].

Inhibition of Coagulation and Influence on Platelet Function

Generally, HMG-CoA reductase inhibitors are highly effective in the prevention of the atherosclerotic vascular disease, especially coronary artery disease. This event has been ascribed to their ability to prevent thrombus formation by modulating the blood coagulation cascade at multiple levels and exerting pro-fibrinolytic and anti-platelet effects. Blood coagulation is a complex process that involves a cascade of proteases and it can be activated through tissue factor (extrinsic pathway) or by contact activation (intrinsic pathway), with both of them culminating in the conversion of prothrombin into thrombin, which catalyses the transformation of fibrinogen in fibrin, forming fibrin-rich clots not only in the veins but also in platelet-rich thrombi typical of the high-flow and high-pressure arterial system [49,52,53].

Tissue factor (TF) is the principal physiological initiator of blood clotting, binding to factor VII/VIIa and activating the extrinsic clotting cascade. It has been demonstrated that simvastatin, in opposition to the hydrophilic pravastatin, decreases the TF mRNA expression and its activity in cultured human monocytes/macrophages obtained from healthy individuals [54]. Importantly, it also revealed to reduce monocyte TF expression in hypercholesterolemic patients [55]. This decrease in TF expression by simvastatin has been found to be, in part, mediated by the inhibition of the activation of NF-kB. Moreover, simvastatin inhibited thrombin-induced TF expression in human aortic endothelial cells, probably by reducing RhoA kinase activation [53]. Moreover, the activity of the tissue factor pathway inhibitor (TFPI), a relevant endogenous factor that inhibits the TF–FVIIa complex, decreases after simvastatin, lovastatin, fluvastatin and atorvastatin administration, potentiating their anti-coagulation effects [53].

Beyond inhibiting plasmatic pathways of thrombus formation, simvastatin also affects the fibrinolytic pathway, which is initiated by the tPA that converts plasminogen to plasmin which, in turn, breaks down the fibrin cap. In mesothelial cells, simvastatin increased tPA expression and suppressed the production of the plasminogen activator inhibitor 1 (PAI-1) that, physiologically, prevents the excessive fibrinolysis. Mechanisms involving geranylgeranyl-modified intermediates and actin skeleton perturbation have been suggested to underline this pleiotropic effect of simvastatin [56].

Finally, simvastatin also deactivates platelets in humans, preventing thrombus formation. The mechanisms suggested for the reduced platelet function under simvastatin treatment include: the up-regulation of simvastatin on eNOS, increasing NO that is known to inhibit the platelet aggregation; the reduction of cholesterol content of platelet membranes [36,38]; the decreased synthesis of thromboxane A2 [36] and the inhibitory effect on Rho-GTPase family [57]. Moreover, it was also found that statins activate the peroxisome proliferator-activated receptors system in platelets, dampening the release of pro-inflammatory/pro-thrombotic mediators and aggregation [58].

Stabilization of Atherosclerotic Plaques

Atherosclerotic lesions integrate several of the aforementioned thrombogenic materials in a lipid core that is separated from bloodstream by a fibrous cap mainly composed of collagen. Weakened fibrous caps lead to plaque instability and rupture, ensuing thrombosis. Reducing lipid levels in plasma, simvastatin may contribute to plaque stability by reducing their size or modifying the physicochemical properties of the lipid core. However, this effect of statins on the plaque size is assessed as minimal in angiography and it tends to occur over an extended time, suggesting that other mechanisms besides lipid lowering are involved. Indeed, it has been clinically evidenced that simvastatin inhibits metalloproteins. Metalloproteins are zinc-dependent proteolytic enzymes, physiologically secreted by activated macrophages, with an important role as weakening agents of the fibrous cap of atherogenic. Their levels are basal, but they are considerably increased in diseases such as multiple sclerosis, ischemic stroke and neurodegenerative pathologies [52,59,60]. By reducing lipids plasma levels and inhibiting metalloproteins independently of cholesterol mechanisms, simvastatin stabilizes plaques, decreasing their size and propensity to rupture [36,61].

Immunomodulatory and Anti-Inflammatory Activities

Statins display a variety of effects on the immune system mainly triggering the major histocompatibility complex (MHC), the leukocyte migration and the cytokine network. Most of the studies show that statins inhibit the activation of the immune response, tissue infiltration by immune cells and inflammation pathways. Although, up to today, no single mechanism has been proposed to explain these activities, several effects seem to depend on the depletion of isoprenoids, specifically GGPP [38].

One of the mechanisms through which statins inhibit the immune response is their interference on the process of antigen presentation. Physiologically, an efficient activation of lymphocyte-T cells is mediated by MHC class II (MHC-II) and CD40/CD40L; indeed, the antigen presenting cells express constitutively MHC-II, while the induction of interferon gamma (IFN-γ) leads to an increase of MHC-II in endothelial cells and monocytes [36]. Statins reduce both the constitutive and induced expression of MHC-II molecules by a GGPP-dependent mechanism, repressing the T-cells activation [62,63]. Particularly for simvastatin, it has been demonstrated that it suppresses T-cell activation and proliferation by Ras pathway [64]. Moreover, in vascular cells, simvastatin emerges as the statin with highest ability to reduce IFN-γ-induced CD40 expression, followed by lovastatin, pravastatin and atorvastatin [65]. The CD40 signalling pathway plays a critical role in the initiation of the immune response by inducing inflammatory responses with secretion of pro-inflammatory cytokines and chemokine. In fact, several studies suggest inhibitory effects of statins on pro-inflammatory cytokine production, including IFN-γ, TNF-α and interleukins in microglia, astrocytes and mononuclear cells. Simvastatin seemed to reduce the levels of IL-6 in microglial cells and it also revealed to reduce the levels of the high-sensitivity C-reactive protein in patients with metabolic syndrome, decreasing, subsequently, the plasma levels of IL-6 and TNF-α [66].

Simvastatin and Bone Metabolism

In a bisphosphonate-like manner, simvastatin inhibits the osteoclasts activation by preventing the mevalonate production that culminates in the disruption of downstream intracellular signalling pathways in osteoclasts. As already herein referred, Rho, Rac and Rab are activated after prenylation; in the osteoclasts this reaction adds the lipid chain that anchors the GTP binding proteins into the membrane of the osteoclasts. This is an essential step for the osteoclasts to form ruffled borders to seal a portion of the bone and promote the release of proteolytic enzymes vesicles that dissolve the underlying bone. Thus, by inhibiting the HMG-CoA reductase, simvastatin inhibits the prenylation of GTP binding proteins, inducing the osteoclast apoptosis and inhibiting osteoclast generation [67,68].

Moreover, and probably because the small GTPase prenylated by-products negatively regulate the expression of the bone morphogenetic protein (BMP) type 2 (BMP-2), simvastatin seems to stimulate the expression of BMP-2, increasing the osteoblast expression, differentiation and, subsequently, enhancing bone formation [45,69,70]. Inducing BMP-2, simvastatin also inhibited adipogenesis [69]; this is important since osteoporosis is accompanied by an unwanted increase in bone marrow adipose tissue. Recently, it has also been demonstrated that simvastatin enhanced the proliferation and recruitment of osteoprogenitor cells, which is a critical step in the early stages of bone healing [71].

Undoubtedly, BMP-2 plays a central role in osteoblast maturation and bone formation induced by simvastatin. Other mechanisms are probably involved including the enhancement of alkaline phosphatase activity and mineralization, the increment of expression of bone sialoprotein, osteocalcin and type I collagen, and the stimulation of vascular endothelial growth factor release in bone tissue which promotes the osteoblast differentiation and bone nodule formation [45].

Since vascular invasion is a prerequisite for calcification during endochondral bone formation and inflammation seems to be responsible for an imbalanced bone metabolism, it is probable that simvastatin increases bone formation and favours the bone resorption due to its well established pro-angiogenic and anti-inflammatory effects [7].

Therapeutic Use of Simvastatin Beyond Hypercholesterolemia: Non-Clinical and Clinical Evidence

The aforementioned evidence supporting the pleiotropic effects of simvastatin clearly suggest a potential use of this drug beyond its lipid lowering properties in several acute and chronic pathologies. Accordingly, the most promising applications of simvastatin in humans seem to be related to its anti-inflammatory, immunomodulatory and anti-coagulant effects. This fact contributed to the conduction of several non-clinical and clinical studies with the aim of assessing the effectiveness of simvastatin in neurological diseases including the Alzheimer's disease, dementia, multiple sclerosis and Parkinson's disease, bone metabolic diseases and cancer treatment. Table 3 summarizes the principal clinical studies developed in these areas and their main results.

Simvastatin in Neurological Diseases

On the basis of its pharmacological properties and in vitro studies, simvastatin was expected to be the most promising candidate amongst the statin drugs for a neuroprotective drug, because of its lipophilicity and higher ability to overcome the BBB.

As observed in Table 3, most of the clinical studies target the oral administration of simvastatin in Alzheimer's disease and dementia. This is a chronic neurodegenerative disorder characterized by brain senile plaques composed of ß-amyloid aggregated forms, cell death of cholinergic neurons, microglial activation and inflammation [98].

Table 3. Summary of the most relevant clinical studies about simvastatin administration in neurological diseases, cancer treatment and bone metabolic diseases

Pathology	Study type	Population	Simvastatin Dose	Other drugs administered	Follow up	Main Results	Reference
Alzheimer's Disease and Dementia	Epidemiological	1364 AD subjects	NS	ATOR, CER, FLU, PRA	6 years	Lower risk of developing dementia.	[72]
	Epidemiological	60,349 AD subjects	NS	LOV, PRA	N/A	Protective effect of LOV and PRA on AD prevalence; No effect with Simvastatin.	[73]
	Clinical trial (Phase III)	20,536 AD subjects	40 mg/day	-	5 years	No differences in cognition.	[74]
	Epidemiological	4895 AD subjects	NS	ATOR, CER, FLU, LOVA, PRA	3 years	No correlation found with the risk of developing dementia or AD.	[75]
	Clinical trial (Phase II)	23 AD subjects	40 mg/day	PRA	14 weeks	Protective effect on AD development.	[76]
	Epidemiological	1021 AD subjects	NS	ATOR, CER, FLU, LOVA, PRA, ROSU	5 years	Reduction of the incidence of dementia and cognitive impairment.	[77]

Pathology	Study type	Population	Simvastatin Dose	Other drugs administered	Follow up	Main Results	Reference
	Epidemiological	929 AD subjects	NS	ATOR, FLU, LOVA, PRA	12 years	Decreased Aß pathological alteration; No effects on AD risk or cognitive ability.	[78]
	Clinical trial (Phase II)	57 AD subjects	40 mg/day	-	4 months	Improved cognitive function in middle-aged adults.	[76]
	Epidemiological	6992 AD subjects	NS	ATOR, CER, FLU, PRA, ROSU	≈9 years	Reduced risk of late-onset AD.	[79]
	Clinical trial (Phase II)	406 AD subjects	20 mg/day (6 weeks); 40 mg/day (> 6 weeks)	-	18 months	No benefits on AD treatment.	[80]
	Population-based, nested case control study	152,729	NS	ATOR, CER, FLU, PRA, ROSU	21 months	Decrease the risk of dementia.	[81]
Multiple Sclerosis	Multi-centre, open-label study	28 patients with RRMS	80 mg/day	-	NS	Reduction of the number (≈44%) and volume (≈41%) of the new GELs.	[82]

Table 3. (Continued)

Pathology	Study type	Population	Simvastatin Dose	Other drugs administered	Follow up	Main Results	Reference
	Prospective Trial	562 patients with RRMS	NS (+ IFN-ß-1a 30µgIM/week)	ATOR, PRA, LOVA, FLU	2 years	No significant differences in the annualized rate of relapse, disability progression, number of GELs, or number of new or enlarging T2 lesions.	[83]
	Clinical Trial	85 patients with RRMS	40 mg/day	-	1 year	In relation to placebo, simvastatin: Reduced the total attack number; Reduced the EDSS; Increased the number of GELs (not considered statistically significant).	[84]
	Clinical Trial (Phase IV)	28 patients with RRMS	80 mg/day (+ IFN-ß-1a 30µgIM/week)	-	NS	No difference in annualized rate of relapse; Development of new T2 lesions.	[85]

Pathology	Study type	Population	Simvastatin Dose	Other drugs administered	Follow up	Main Results	Reference
	Double-blind controlled clinical trial	140 patients with secondary progressive multiple sclerosis	80 mg/day	-	2 years	Simvastatin reduced the annualized rate of whole-brain atrophy compared with placebo, and was well tolerated and safe.	[86]
Dementia and Parkinson's Disease	Observational	700,000 patients, aged ≥65 years, taking simvastatin and not diagnosis with AD or PD	NS	-	-	Significant reduction in the incidence of dementia and PD.	[87]
Parkinson's Disease	Observational	43,810 statin initiators PD-free		NS	-	Continuation of simvastatin therapy was associated to a decreased in PD incidence compared to discontinuation users.	[88]
Cancer diseases	Open nonrandomized pilot study	10 patients with untreated B-cell chronic lymphocytic leukemia	40 mg/day	-	12 weeks	No significant change in clinical disease status during the treatment; 40% of the patients developed progressive disease	[89]

Table 3. (Continued)

Pathology	Study type	Population	Simvastatin Dose	Other drugs administered	Follow up	Main Results	Reference
						during the subsequent year and 60% within 2 years after stopping simvastatin.	
	Clinical Trial (Phase II)	49 patients with metastatic adenocarcinoma of rectum colon	40 mg/day (+ FOLFIRI)	-	NS	Response rate and median survival time similar to those with FOLFIRI alone; Prolonged time to progression compared with FOLFIRI alone.	[90]
Bone diseases	Observational	53 individuals	20 mg/day	-	4 weeks	Increased serum osteocalcin	[91]
	Controlled trial	85 women	20 -40 mg/day	-	12 weeks	Decreased bone specific serum alkaline phosphatase.	[92]
	Prospective cohort	30 postmenopausal hypercholesterolemic women	40 mg/day	-	12 months	Increased bone specific serum alkaline phosphatase.	[93]

Pathology	Study type	Population	Simvastatin Dose	Other drugs administered	Follow up	Main Results	Reference
	Clinical Trial	4444 individuals taking simvastatin; 19% with heart disease	20-40 mg/day	-	5.5 years	No beneficial effect on risk of fractures.	[94]
	Observational	37 women with Diabetes *Mellitus* 2	NS	-	NS	No significant increase on BMD.	[95]
	Prospective randomized control trial	62 patients	20 mg/day	-	12 weeks	No significant alterations on BMD.	[96]
	Prospective randomized control trial	212 patients with osteopenia and hypercholesterolemia	40-80 mg/day	-	18 months	Increase of BMD; Increase of bone formation; Reduction of bone resorption.	[97]

Aß, Alzheimer's amyloid peptide; AD, Alzheimer's disease; ATOR, atorvastatin; BMD, bone mineral density; CER, Cerivastatin; EDSS, Expanded Disability Status Scale scores; FLU, fluvastatin; FOLFIRI, folinic acid/5-fluorouracil/irinotecan; GELs, gadolinium-enhancing lesions; IFN, Interferon; LOVA, lovastatin; MRI, magnetic resonance imaging; NS, not specified; PD, Parkinson's Disease; PRA, pravastatin; ROS, rosuvastatin; RRMS, Relapsing remitting multiple sclerosis.

The link between Alzheimer's disease and hypercholesterolemia has been explored for almost two decades, suggesting that an elevated serum cholesterol level is a risk factor for the pathology development [99]. The high intracellular cholesterol levels promote the production of Alzheimer's amyloid (Aß) peptide, by shifting the cleavage of amyloid precursor protein from α to ß [7]; moreover it has also been associated to the apoε4 allele of apolipoprotein E gene, which is the major risk factor for Alzheimer's disease. In vitro studies in several cell lines and in vivo pre-clinical studies revealed that simvastatin reduces Aß levels, probably by inhibiting prenylation of Rab family protein (which function is associated with Aß production) and reduction of the Rho GTPase protein expression, with consequent decrease of Aß secretion and Aß-induced inflammation [100-102]. It is noteworthy that the beneficial effects of statins on neuroinflammation and neurodegeneration have also been reported in other disease animal models besides Alzheimer's disease where simvastatin demonstrated to attenuate learning and memory impairment in mice without affecting brain Aß levels [103].

In spite of the increasing evidence of in vitro and in vivo animal models suggests a promissory neuroprotective effect of simvastatin on the onset and progression of Alzheimer's disease and dementia [17,37,76,104], clinical evidence is not so linear (Table 3). The first epidemiological evidence on the beneficial effect of several statins, including simvastatin, in lowering the risk of developing dementia was found in 2000 by Jick et al. [72]. However, in the same year, Wolozin et al. [73] showed that simvastatin was not associated to a reduced Alzheimer's disease prevalence, in opposition to lovastatin and pravastatin. Similar results were found in another epidemiological study [75], while the results from the Sacramento Area Latino Study on Aging (SALSA), a prospective cohort observational study, indicated that statins (atorvastatin, cerivastatin, fluvastatin, lovastatin, pravastatin, rosuvastatin and simvastatin analyzed together) were associated with a significant reduction in the incidence of combined dementia and cognitive impairment without dementia; furthermore, the results of the Rotterdam Study, a prospective study involving a cohort of almost 7000 subjects, found that statins (atorvastatin, cerivastatin, fluvastatin, pravastatin, rosuvastatin and simvastatin analyzed together and simvastatin and pravastatin analyzed separately) correlate with almost 50% of reduced risk of late-onset Alzheimer's disease [79].

These observational studies generated initial enthusiasm for statins as preventive agents for Alzheimer's disease and dementia development, and several randomized clinical trials were planned in order to support their neuroprotective activity (Table 3). Favourable results were obtained by

Carlsson et al. [105] who reported that simvastatin (40 mg/day) improved cognitive function in middle-aged adults whose parents suffered from Alzheimer's disease; this hypothesis was also supported by the findings of a clinical study in which hypercholesterolemic subjects without dementia were administered simvastatin (40 mg/day) or pravastatin (80 mg/day) for 14 weeks [76]. However, the recent Cholesterol-Lowering Agent to Slow the Progression of Alzheimer's disease trial (CLASP-AD), a multicenter, randomized, double-blind, placebo-controlled phase II trial, with the aim of investigating effects of simvastatin treatment for 18 months (20 mg/day for 6 weeks, then 40 mg/day for the remainder of the study period) versus placebo [80,106], found that simvastatin had no positive effect on the Alzheimer's disease treatment. Several experimental factors, such as the subject selection criteria, the stage of the disease and the duration of treatment could in part explain the divergence among different studies and should be taken into account to evaluate statins effectiveness on Alzheimer's disease onset and progression.

Nevertheless, the aforementioned findings also address a protective role of simvastatin in preventing cognitive decline in non-Alzheimer's disease-related and suggest potential therapeutic applications in other chronic inflammatory disorders of the CNS, namely the multiple sclerosis. Classic multiple sclerosis lesions, often denoted T2 hyperintensity lesions, are the most associated with the "relapses" in the disease. Because of the immunomodulatory activity of simvastatin, this drug is under investigation as a treatment for multiple sclerosis. Indeed, until now, few studies enrolling a limited number of patients argued that simvastatin diminished the relapses and the number of gadolinium-enhancing lesions (GELs) in relapsing-remitting multiple sclerosis (MMRS) (Table 3). However these encouraging results need to be interpreted cautiously, particularly when analyzing the prospective study developed by Rudick and collaborators [83] and the SIMCOMBIN clinical trial (phase IV) which reported no differences in annualized rate of relapse and, even, an increase of T2 lesions (Table 3).

Interestingly, statins do not worsen Parkinson's disease and, in fact, they seem to reduce the inflammation process that contributes to the aetiology of Parkinson's disease. Both in vivo studies performed in animals [38,42,107] and in humans [87,88] demonstrated that simvastatin may be beneficial to prevent Parkinson's disease. The observational studies clearly outline that simvastatin reduces significantly the incidence of dementia and Parkinson's disease in patients taking simvastatin, and initially not diagnosed with Parkinson's disease (Table 3).

Simvastatin in Cancer Therapy

As described throughout the section "Pleiotropic effects of simvastatin" of the present chapter, simvastatin shows anti-proliferative, anti-apoptotic and anti-invasive effects that may support an eventual success as a chemotherapeutic drug. The anticancer potential of simvastatin has been investigated in vitro and in animal models as recently reviewed by Gazzerro et al. [7]. However, to the best of our knowledge, there are only two clinical trials that investigated the effect of simvastatin in two distinct cancer types, the metastatic adenocarcinoma of rectum or colon [89,90] and the B-cell chronic lymphocytic leukaemia [89].

Simvastatin has been tested in combination with folinic acid/5-fluorouracil/irinotecan (FOLFIRI), a conventional second-line therapy used in colorectal cancer, and the overall responsive rate and the median survival of the patients were similar to that obtained with FOLFIRI alone. Moreover, the simvastatin combined with irinotecan induced a slight increase in the time to progression, without increasing the toxicity (Table 3) and therefore it was suggested to be co-administered with anti-inflammatory drugs [108]. Simvastatin was also tested in 10 patients affected with chronic lymphocytic leukaemia, with no significant changes in the clinical disease status and 40% of the patients experienced a progression of the neoplasia during the subsequent year (Table 3).

Simvastatin in Bone Diseases

The in vitro and in vivo non-clinical discovery of statins as bone metabolic agents led to the development of several studies to evaluate the clinical utility of statins with respect to bone health. The main objectives were to assess the influence of statins on fracture risk, bone mineral density and biochemical markers of bone metabolism [92]. Most of the studies are observational and several of them evaluated the effect of statins in general, without presenting the results separately for each statin in particular [109-111]. Because, in these studies, data interpretation specifically for simvastatin is hampered, Table 3 presents the main clinical studies with results that pertain only to simvastatin. Most of the studies based on either measurement of bone mineral density (BMD), fracture risk or biochemical markers of bone metabolism, comprising markers for bone formation (e.g. osteocalcin, bone specific alkaline phosphatase), which serve as a tool for the diagnosis of osteoporosis and have been studied to assess the potential of simvastatin in the treatment of osteoporosis (Table 3).

Association between statins use and risk fracture is a contentious issue. The Scandinavian Simvastatin Survival Study (4S), which analyzed the fracture risk in simvastatin-treated and placebo groups, reported no beneficial effects on the risk of fractures (Table 3). In turn, the recent prospective randomized control trial study enrolling 212 patients with hyperlipidaemia and osteopenia deserves particular attention in view of the positive effect of simvastatin to significantly increase BMD and bone markers, supporting an increase in bone formation and a reduction of bone resorption [97]. In a similar way to the remaining clinical studies summarized in Table 3, this study also suffers from some limitations and confounders that do not clarify whether simvastatin is in fact beneficial in preventing and/or slowing bone loss in the aging osteoporotic population.

One of the drawbacks that have been hypothesized for the clinical failure and discrepant results of simvastatin in bone diseases is the low bone specificity of this drug [92]. Indeed, the minimal concentration of simvastatin required to have beneficial action on bone is a critical need in exploring its action as anti-osteoporotic agent. Therefore, several formulations have been developed and tested in animals in an attempt to delivering simvastatin specifically to the bone. An almost 50% increase in new bone formation was observed after only five days of treatment when simvastatin was injected into the subcutaneous tissue overlying the calvaria of mice [112]. A matrix controlled delivery system of simvastatin besides reducing the dose and dosage frequency, promoted a 53% increase at the thickest point of the calvarial bone [113].

Finally, it should be emphasized that, when targeting simvastatin to the bone, the desired effects can be achieved at lower doses and this has been one of the aspects focused in recent research [114].

Conclusion

In addition to its potent cardio-protective and anti-atherosclerotic effects as a result of its ability to reduce endogenous cholesterol synthesis, simvastatin is currently being considered for medical conditions beyond cardiovascular diseases. Indeed, compelling in vitro and in vivo non-clinical studies support pleiotropic effects of simvastatin related to its ability to regulate NO bioavailability, to improve the endothelial function and to regulate cell proliferation and bone metabolism; in addition, its antioxidant, immunomodulatory and anti-inflammatory effects are currently unquestionable. Although a significant amount of non-clinical data support these findings, pleiotropic action of simvastatin remains an evolving concept because some conflicting results have been obtained in clinical studies. Nevertheless, it is apparent that most patients with CNS disease, bone disease or cancer probably benefit to some extent from therapy with simvastatin. Thus, further research is still needed to determine the optimal therapeutic threshold, type of administration formulation and clinical effectiveness.

References

[1] Cholesterol Treatment Trialists' (CTT) Collaborators. Efficacy and safety of cholesterol-lowering treatment: prospective meta-analysis of data from 90,056 participants in 14 randomised trials of statins. *Lancet.* 2005; 366(9493): 1267-78.

[2] Law MR, Wald NJ, Rudnicka AR. Quantifying effect of statins on low density lipoprotein cholesterol, ischaemic heart disease, and stroke: systematic review and meta-analysis. *Vasc. Med.* 2003; 8(4): 289-290.

[3] Zhou Q, Liao JK. Pleiotropic effects of statins. – Basic research and clinical perspectives. *Cir. J.* 2010; 74(5): 818-826.

[4] Food and Drug Administration, FDA Drug Safety Communication: New restrictions, contraindications, and dose limitations for Zocor (simvastatin) to reduce the risk of muscle injury. 2011. Available at http://www.fda.gov/Drugs/DrugSafety/ucm256581.htm

[5] Walker R, Williams H. Dyslipidaemia. Clinical Pharmacy and Therapeutics, ed. Walker, R. and Wittlesea C., 2012, 5th ed., Churchill Livingstone, *Elsevier,* 389-411.

[6] Gouni-Berthold I, et al. Effects of ezetimibe and/or simvastatin on LDL receptor protein expression and on LDL receptor and HMG-CoA reductase gene expression: A randomized trial in healthy men. *Atherosclerosis.* 2008; 198(1): 198-207.

[7] Gazzerro, et al. Pharmacological Actions of Statins: A Critical Appraisal in the Management of Cancer. Pharmacol Rev. 2012; 64(1): 102-146.

[8] Kajinami K, Takekoshi N, Saito Y. Pitavastatin: Efficacy and Safety Profiles of A Novel Synthetic HMG-CoA Reductase Inhibitor. Cardiovasc Drug Rev. 2003; 21(3): 199-215.

[9] Mukhtar RY, Reid J, Reckless JP. Pitavastatin. *Int J Clin Pract.* 2005; 59(2): 239-252.
[10] Saito Y. Critical appraisal of the role of pitavastatin in treating dyslipidemias and achieving lipid goals. *Vasc Health Risk Mang.* 2009; 5: 921-936.
[11] Schachter M. Chemical, pharmacokinetic and pharmacodynamic properties of statins: an update. *Fundam Clin Pharmacol.* 2005; 19(1): 117-125.
[12] Merck Sharp & Dohme Ltd. Zocor (Simvastatin tablets) Prescribing Information. 2014. Available at http://www.merck.com/product/usa/pi_circulars/z/zocor/zocor_pi.pdf
[13] Istvan ES, Deisenhofer J. Structural Mechanism for Statin Inhibition of HMG-CoA Reductase. *Science.* 2001; 292(5519): 1160-1164.
[14] Davidson, MH. Rosuvastatin: a highly efficacious statin for the treatment of dyslipidaemia. *Expert Opin Investig Drugs.* 2002; 11(3): 125-141.
[15] Toth PP; Dayspring, TD. Drug safety evaluation of rosuvastatin. *Expert Opin Drug Saf.* 2011; 10(6): 969-986.
[16] Corsini A, et al. New insights into the pharmacodynamic and pharmacokinetic properties of statins. *Pharmacol Ther.* 1999; 84(3): 413-428.
[17] Shepardson NE, Shankar GM, Selkoe DJ. Cholesterol Level and Statin Use in Alzheimer Disease: I. Review of epidemiological and preclinical studies. *Arch Neurol.* 2011; 68(10): 1239-1244.
[18] Cheng H, et al. Influence of age and gender on the plasma profiles of 3-hydroxy-3-methylglutaryl-coenzyme A (HMG-CoA) reductase inhibitory activity following multiple doses of lovastatin and simvastatin. *Pharmac Res.* 1992; 9(12): 1629-1633.
[19] Prueksaritanont T, Ma B, Yu N. The human hepatic metabolism of simvastatin hydroxy acid is mediated primarily by CYP3A, and not CYP2D6. *Br J Clin Pharmacol.* 2003; 56(1): 120-124.
[20] McKenney JM. Pharmacologic characteristics of statins. *Clin Cardiol.* 2003; 26(Suppl III): III-32-III-38.
[21] Saheki A, et al. In vivo and in vitro blood-brain barrier transporter of 3-hydroxy-3-methylglutaryl coenzyme A (HMG-CoA) reductase inhibitors. *Pharmac Res.* 1994; 11(2): 305-311.
[22] Shitara Y, Sugiyama Y. Pharmacokinetic and pharmacodynamic alterations of 3-hydroxy-3-methylglutaryl coenzyme A (HMG-CoA) reductase inhibitors: Drug–drug interactions and interindividual

differences in transporter and metabolic enzyme functions. *Pharmacol Ther.* 2006; 112(1): 71-105.

[23] Armitage J. The safety of statins in clinical practice. *Lancet.* 2007; 370(9601): 1781-1790.

[24] Lemos JA, et al. Early Intensive vs a Delayed Conservative Simvastatin Strategy in Patients With Acute Coronary Syndromes: phase Z of the A to Z trial. *JAMA.* 2004; 292(11): 1307-1316.

[25] Jacobson TA. Comparative Pharmacokinetic Interaction Profiles of Pravastatin, Simvastatin, and Atorvastatin When Coadministered With Cytochrome P450 Inhibitors. *Am J Cardiol.* 2004; 94(9): 1140-1146.

[26] Florentin M, Elisaf MS. Simvastatin interactions with other drugs. *Expert Opin Drug Saf.* 2012; 11(3): 439-444.

[27] Neuvonen PJ, Kantola T, Kivistö KT. Simvastatin but not pravastatin is very susceptible to interaction with the CYP3A4 inhibitor itraconazole. Clin Pharmacol Ther. 1998; 63(3): 332-341.

[28] Burtenshaw AJ, Sellors G, Downing R. Presumed interaction of fusidic acid with simvastatin. *Anaesthesia.* 2008; 63(6): 656-658.

[29] Hsyu P-H, et al. Pharmacokinetic Interactions between Nelfinavir and 3-Hydroxy-3-Methylglutaryl Coenzyme A Reductase Inhibitors Atorvastatin and Simvastatin. *Antimicrob Agents Chemother.* 2001; 45(12): 3445-3450.

[30] Zhang R, et al. Rhabdomyolysis induced by simvastatin-diltiazem interaction in unrecognized hypothyroidism. *J Geriat Cardiol.* 2010; 7(2):126-128.

[31] Hickmott H, Wynne H, Kamali F. The effect of simvastatin co-medication on warfarin anticoagulation response and dose requirements. *Thromb Haemost.* 2003; 89(5): 949-950.

[32] Ucar M, et al. Carbamazepine markedly reduces serum concentrations of simvastatin and simvastatin acid. *Eur J Clin Pharmacol.* 2004; 59(12): 879-882.

[33] Xu Y, et al. Simulation of Clinical Drug-Drug Interactions from Hepatocyte CYP3A4 Induction Data and Its Potential Utility in Trial Designs. *Drug Metab Dispos.* 2011; 39(7): 1139-1148.

[34] Davignon J. Beneficial Cardiovascular Pleiotropic Effects of Statins. *Circulation.* 2004; 109(Suppl 1): III39-III43.

[35] Gomez SI, et al. The pleiotropic effects of the hydroxy-methyl-glutaryl-CoA reductase inhibitors in renal disease. *Int J Nephrol Renovas Dis.* 2014; 7: 123-130.

[36] Liao JK, Laufs U. Pleiotropic effects of statins. *Annu Rev Pharmacol Toxicol.* 2005; 45: 98-118.

[37] Reiss AB, Wirkowski E. Statins in neurological disorders: mechanisms and therapeutic value. *Scientific World Journal.* 2009; 9: 1242-1259.

[38] Most PJ, et al. Statins: Mechanisms of neuroprotection. *Prog Meurobiol* 2009; 88(1): 64-75.

[39] Kosmidou I, et al. Statin treatment and 3'polyadenylation of eNOS mRNA. *Arterioscler Thromb Vasc Biol.* 2007; 27(12): 2642-2649.

[40] Laufs U, et al. Suppression of endothelial nitric oxide production after withdrawal of statin treatment is mediated by negative feedback regulation of rho GTPase gene transcription. *Circulation.* 2000; 102(25): 3104-3110.

[41] Guzik TJ, Harrison DG. Vascular NADPH oxidases as drug targets for novel antioxidant strategies. *Drug Discov Today.* 2006; 11(11-12): 524-533.

[42] Malfitano AM, et al. Statins in neurological disorders: an overview and update. *Pharmacol Res.* 2014; 88: 74-83.

[43] Morikawa S, et al. The effect of statins on mRNS levels of genes related to inflammation, coagulation, and vascular constriction in HUVEC. *J Atheroscler Thromb.* 2002; 9(4): 178-183.

[44] Kureishi Y, et al. The HMG-CoA reductase inhibitor simvastatin activates the protein kinase Akt and promotes angiogenesis in normocholesterolemic animals. *Nat Med.* 2000; 6(9): 1004-1010.

[45] Park H-J, et al. 3-Hydroxy-3-Methylglutaryl Coenzyme A Reductase Inhibitors Interfere With Angiogenesis by Inhibiting the Geranylgeranylation of RhoA. *Circ Res.* 2002; 91(2): 143-150.

[46] Szmitko PE, et al. Endothelial Progenitor Cells New Hope for a Broken Heart. *Circulation.* 2003; 107(24): 3093-3100.

[47] Urbich C, Dimmeler S. Endothelial progenitor cells: characterization and role in vascular biology. *Circ Res.* 2004; 95(4): 343-353.

[48] Walter D, et al. Statin Therapy Accelerates Reendothelialization A Novel Effect Involving Mobilization and Incorporation of Bone Marrow–Derived Endothelial Progenitor Cells. *Circulation.* 2002; 105(25): 3017-3024.

[49] Katsiki N, et al. Effect of HMG-CoA reductase inhibitors on vascular cell apoptosis: Beneficial or detrimental? *Atherosclerosis.* 2010; 211(1): 9-14.

[50] Tang D, et al. Simvastatin potentiates tumor necrosis factor α-mediated apoptosis of human vascular endothelial cells via the inhibition of the geranylgeranylation of RhoA. *Life Sci.* 2006; 79(15): 1484-1492.

[51] Miyashita Y, et al. Oxysterol-induced apoptosis of vascular smooth cells is reduced by HMG-CoA reductase inhibitor, pravastatin. *J Atheroscler Thromb.* 2002; 9(1):65-71.

[52] Rosenberg GA. Matrix metalloproteinases and their multiple roles in neurodegenerative diseases. *Lancet Neurol.* 2009; 8(2): 205-216.

[53] Undas A, Brummel-Ziedins KE, Mann KG. Statins and Blood Coagulation. *Arterioscler Thromb Vasc Biol.* 2005; 25(2): 287-294.

[54] Colli S, et al. Vastatins Inhibit Tissue Factor in Cultured Human Macrophages A Novel Mechanism of Protection Against Atherothrombosis. Arterioscler Throm Vasc Biol. 1997; 17(2): 265-272.

[55] Owens AP, Byrnes JR, Mackman N. Hyperlipidemia, tissuefactor, coagulation, andsimvastatin. *Trends Cardiovasc Med.* 2014; 24(3): 95-98.

[56] Haslinger B, et al. Simvastatin increases fibrinolytic activity in human peritoneal mesothelial cells independent of cholesterol lowering. *Kideny Int.* 2002; 62(5):1611-1619.

[57] Kaneider NC, et al. Rho-GTPase-Dependent Platelet-Neutrophil Interaction Affected by HMG-CoA reductase inhibition with altered adenosine nucleotide release and function. *Arterioscler Thromb Vasc Biol.* 2002; 22(6): 1029-1035.

[58] Ali FY, et al. Antiplatelet Actions of Statins and Fibrates Are Mediated by PPARs. *Arterioscler Thromb Vasc Biol.* 2009; 29(5): 706-711.

[59] Montaner J, et al. Matrix metalloproteinase expression is related to hemorrhagic transformation after cardioembolic stroke. *Stroke.* 2001; 32(12):2762-2767.

[60] Yong VW, et al. Elevation of matrix metalloproteinases (MMPs) in multiple sclerosis and impact of immunomodulators. *J Neurol Sci.* 2007; 259(1-2): 79-84.

[61] Wang S, et al. Reduction of Tissue Plasminogen Activator-Induced Matrix Metalloproteinase-9 by simvastatin in astrocytes. *Stroke.* 2006; 37(7): 1910-1912.

[62] Kuipers HF, et al. Statins Affect Cell-Surface Expression of Major Histocompatibility Complex Class II Molecules by Disrupting Cholesterol-Containing Microdomains. *Hum Immunol.* 2005; 66(6):653-665.

[63] Kuipers HF, Elsen PJ. Immunomodulation by statins: Inhibition of cholesterol vs. isoprenoid biosynthesis. *Biomed Pharmacother.* 2007; 61(7):400-407.

[64] Ghittoni R, et al. Simvastatin inhibits T-cell activation by selectively impairing the function of Ras superfamily GTPases. *FASEB J.* 2005; 19(6): 605-607.

[65] Mulhaupt F, et al. Statins (HMG-CoA reductase inhibitors) reduce CD40 expression in human vascular cells. *Cardiovasc Res.* 2003; 59(3): 755-766.

[66] Jaiswal SR, Sontakk SD. Experimental evaluation of analgesic and ani-inflammatory activity of simvastatin and atorvastatin. *Indian J Pharmacol.* 2012; 44(4): 475-479.

[67] Dunford JE, et al. Inhibition of Protein Prenylation by Bisphosphonates Causes Sustained Activation of Rac, Cdc42, and Rho GTPases. *J Bone Miner Res.* 2006; 21(5): 684-694.

[68] Hughes A, et al. A Comparison between the Effects of Hydrophobic and Hydrophilic Statins on Osteoclast Function In Vitro and Ovariectomy-Induced Bone Loss In Vivo. *Calcif Tissue Int.* 2007; 81(5): 403-413.

[69] Song C, et al. Simvastatin induces osteoblastic differentiation and inhibits adipocytic differentiation in mouse bone marrow stromal cells. *Biochem Biophys Res Commun* 2003; 308(3):458-462.~

[70] Sugiyama M, et al. Compactin and Simvastatin, but Not Pravastatin, Induce Bone Morphogenetic Protein-2 in Human Osteosarcoma Cells. *Biochem Biophys Res Commun.* 2000; 271(3):688-692.

[71] Nyan M, et al. Molecular and Tissue Responses in the Healing of Rat Calvarial Defects After Local Application of Simvastatin Combined With Alpha Tricalcium Phosphate. *J Biomed Res B Appl Biomater.* 2010; 93(1): 65-73.

[72] Jick H, et al. Statins and the risk of dementia. *Lancet.* 2000; 356(9242): 1627-1631.

[73] Wolozin B, et al. Decreased prevalence of Alzheimer disease associated with 3-hydroxy-3-methylglutaryl Coenzyme A reductase inhibitors. *Arch Neurol.* 2000; 57(10): 1439-1443.

[74] Heart Protection Study Collaborative Group. MRC/BHF Heart Protection Study of cholesterol lowering with simvastatin in 20 536 high-risk individuals: a randomised placebocontrolled trial. *Lancet.* 2002; 360(9326): 7-22.

[75] Zandi PP, et al. Do Statins Reduce Risk of Incident Dementia and Alzheimer Disease? *Arch Gen Psychiatry.* 2005; 62(2): 217-224.

[76] Barone E, Di Domenico F, Butterfield DA. Statins more than cholesterol lowering agents in Alzheimer disease: Their pleiotropic functions as potential therapeutic targets. *Biochem Pharmacol.* 2014; 88(4): 605-616.

[77] Cramer C, et al. Use of statins and incidence of dementia and cognitive impairment without dementia in a cohort study. *Neurology.* 2008; 71(5): 344-350.

[78] Rea TD, et al. Statin Use and the Risk of Incident Dementia The Cardiovascular Health Study. *Arch Neurol.* 2005; 62(7): 1047-1051.

[79] Haag MDM, et al. Statins are associated with a reduced risk of Alzheimer disease regardless of lipophilicity. The Rotterdam Study. *J neurol Neurosurg Psychiatry.* 2009; 80(1): 13-17.

[80] Sano M, et al. A randomized, double-blind placebo-controlled trial of simvastatin to treat Alzheimer disease. *Neurology.* 2011; 77(6): 556-563.

[81] Corrao G, et al. Long-term use of statins reduces the risk of hospitalization for dementia. *Atherosclerosis.* 2013; 230(2): 171-176.

[82] Vollmer T, et al. Oral simvastatin treatment in relapsing-remitting multiple sclerosis. *Lancet.* 2004; 369(9421): 1607-1608.

[83] Rudick RA, et al. Effect of statins on clinical and molecular responses to intramuscular interferon beta-1a. *Neurology.* 2009; 72(23):1989-1993.

[84] Togha M, et al. Simvastatin treatment in patients with relapsing-remitting multiple sclerosis receiving interferon beta1a: a double-blind randomized controlled trial. *Mult Scler.* 2010; 16(7): 848-854.

[85] Sorensen PS, et al. Simvastatin as add-on therapy to interferon beta-1a for relapsing-remitting multiple sclerosis (SIMCOMBIN study): a placebo-controlled randomised phase 4 trial. *Lancet Neurol.* 2011; 10(8): 691-701.

[86] Chataway J, et al. Effect of high-dose simvastatin on brain atrophy and disability in secondary progressive multiple sclerosis (MS-STAT): a randomised, placebo-controlled, phase 2 trial. *Lancet.* 2014; 383(9936): 2213-2221.

[87] Wolozin B, et al. Simvastatin is associated with a reduced incidence of dementia and Parkinson's disease. *BMC Med.* 2007; 19: 5-20.

[88] Lee YC, et al. Discontinuation of statin therapy associates with Parkinson disease: a population-based study. *Neurology.* 2013; 81(5): 410-416.

[89] Vitols S, Angelin B, Juliusson G. Simvastatin Impairs mitogen-induced proliferation of malignant B-lymphocytes from humans—in vitro and in vivo studies. *Lipids.* 1997; 32(3):255-262.

[90] Lee J, et al. Simvastatin plus irinotecan, 5-fluorouracil, and leucovorin (FOLFIRI) as first-line chemotherapy in metastatic colorectal patients: a multicenter phase II study. *Cancer Chemother Pharmacol.* 2009; 64(4): 657-663.

[91] Chan M, et al. Simvastatin increases serum osteocalcin concentration in patients treated for hypercholesterolaemia. *J Clin Endoc Metab.* 2001; 86(9): 4556-4559.

[92] Jadhav SB, Jain GK. Statins and osteoporosis: new role for old drugs. *J Pharm Pharmacol.* 2006; 58(1): 3-18.

[93] Montagnani A, et al. Effect of simvastatin treatment on bone mineral density and bone turnover in hypercholesterolemic postmenopausal women: a 1-year longitudinal study. *Bone.* 2003; 32(4): 427-433.

[94] Pedersen TR, et al. Randomised trial of cholesterol lowering in 4444 patients with coronary heart disease: the Scandinavian Simvastatin Survival Study (4S). *Atherosclerosis Suppl.* 2004; 5: 81-87.

[95] Uysal AR, et al. Effect of simvastatin use on bone mineral density in women with type 2 diabetes. *Endocr Pract.* 2007; 13(2): 114-116.

[96] Patil S, et al. Prospective, Double Blind, Randomized, Controlled Trial of Simvastatin in Human Fracture Healing. *J Orthop Res.* 2009; 27(3): 281-285.

[97] Chuengsamarn S, et al. Effects of statins vs. non-statin lipid-lowering therapy on bone formation and bone mineral density biomarkers in patients with hyperlipidemia. *Bone.* 2010; 46(4): 1011-1015.

[98] Humpel C. Chronic mild cerebrovascular dysfunction as a cause for Alzheimer's disease? *Exp Gerontol.* 2011; 46(4):225-232.

[99] Ricciarelli R, et al. Cholesterol and Alzheimer's Disease: A Still Poorly Understood Correlation. *IUBMB Life.* 2012; 64(12):931-935.

[100] Cordle A, et al. Mechanisms of Statin-mediated Inhibition of Small G-protein Function. *J Biol Chem.* 2005; 280(40): 34202-34209.

[101] Fassbender K, et al. Simvastatin strongly reduces levels of Alzheimer's disease beta-amyloid peptides Abeta 42 and Abeta 40 in vitro and in vivo. *Proc Natl Acad Sci USA.* 2001; 98(10): 5856-5861.

[102] Ostrowski SM, et al. Statins reduce amyloid-ß production through inhibition of protein isoprenylation. *J Biol Chem.* 2007; 282(37): 26832-26844.

[103] Li L. Et al. Simvastatin Enhances Learning and Memory Independent of Amyloid Load in Mice. *Ann Neurol.* 2006; 60(6): 729-739.

[104] Sánchez-Ferro A, et al. A review of the potential therapeutic role of statins in the treatment of Alzheimer's disease: current research and opinion. *Neuropsychiatr Dis Treat.* 2013; 9: 55-63.
[105] Carlsson CM, et al. Effects of Simvastatin on Cerebrospinal Fluid Biomarkers and Cognition in Middle-Aged Adults at Risk for Alzheimer's Disease. *J Alzheimers Dis*. 2008; 13(2): 187-197.
[106] Pressman P, Gottfried JA. Journal Club: A randomized, double-blind, placebo-controlled trial of simvastatin to treat Alzheimer disease. *Neurology.* 2012; 79(4): e33-e36.
[107] Roy A, Pahan K. Prospects of statins in Parkinson Disease. *Neuroscientist.* 2011; 17(3): 244-255.
[108] Künzl M, Wasinger C, Hohenegger M. Statins role in cancer prevention and development-recent meta-analyses. *World J Pharmacol.* 2013; 2(4): 100-106.
[109] Bauer DC, et al. Use of statins and fracture. *Arch Intern Med.* 2004; 164: 146-152.
[110] Gonyeau MJ, Statins and Osteoporosis: A Clinical Review. *Pharmacotherapy.* 2005; 25(2): 228-243.
[111] Uzzan B, et al. Effects of statins on bone mineral density: A meta-analysis of clinical studies. *Bone.* 2007; 40(6): 1581-1587.
[112] Mundy G, et al. Stimulation of Bone Formation in Vitro and in Rodents by Statins. *Science.* 1999; 286(5446):1946-1949.
[113] Thylin MR, et al. Effects of simvastatin gels on murine calvarial bone. *J Periodontol.* 2002; 73(10):1141-1148.
[114] Pauly, S., et al., Simvastatin locally applied from a biodegradable coating of osteosynthetic implants improves fracture healing comparable to BMP-2 application. *Bone,* 2009. 45(3): p. 505-511.

In: Simvastatin Delivery
Editors: Alberto A. C. C. Pais et al.
ISBN: 978-1-63482-148-3

Chapter 3

Crossing the Skin Barrier: A Development Strategy

Carla Vitorino[1,2*], António Almeida[3], João José Sousa[1,2] and Alberto Pais[4]

[1] Laboratory of Pharmacology, Faculty of Pharmacy, University of Coimbra, Pólo das Ciências da Saúde, Azinhaga de Santa Comba, Coimbra, Portugal
[2] CNC – Centre for Neuroscience and Cell Biology, University of Coimbra, Coimbra, Portugal
[3] CICS-UBI – Health Sciences Research Centre, University of Beira Interior, Covilhã, Portugal

Abstract

This chapter describes the development of a transdermal delivery system for the simultaneous administration of simvastatin and olanzapine.

In order to overcome the barrier imposed by the stratum corneum (SC), the outermost layer of the skin, the combination of lipid nanoparticles and chemical enhancers is addressed, in the perspective of passive strategies. Additionally, the active microneedle-mediated delivery of nanoparticles into the skin is investigated as an alternative to potentiate

* Laboratory of Pharmaceutical Technology, Faculty of Pharmacy, University of Coimbra, Pólo das Ciências da Saúde, Azinhaga de Santa Comba, 3000-548 Coimbra, Portugal; Email: csvitorino@ff.uc.pt.

drug transport. Lipid nanoparticles, comprising solid lipid nanoparticles (SLN) and nanostructured lipid carriers (NLC) were prepared by the solvent emulsification-evaporation (SE/E) and high pressure homogenization (HPH) methods. Full factorial designs, 2^k, were conducted to rationalize and optimize formulation composition, production conditions and application. The combined effect of lipid nanoparticles and chemical enhancers was investigated by *in vitro*, *in silico* and cellular viability methodologies. The formulations were assessed in a joint *in vitro/in vivo* approach.

As a result of the reduced solubility of olanzapine in the solid lipid, tripalmitin, NLC were selected for co-encapsulation. In what pertains to NLC production, the HPH technique was chosen, since it allowed a higher drug loading, a more sustained release, better permeation rate, in conjunction with the ability to scale up, avoidance of organic solvents and shorter production times.

The *in vitro* skin experiments showed that the external medium in the NLC dispersion strongly influenced permeation. Moreover, it was also seen that the use of NLC determined a synergistic effect with the selected permeation enhancers, ethanol and limonene, thus promoting marked flux enhancement ratios, relative to the drugs in solution. Converting the formulation into a gel reduced the flow rate. A correlation between enhancer positioning in the lipid bilayer and enhancement effect was suggested from molecular dynamics studies that corroborated the experimental results.

A study, focusing on rheological, mechanical and physicochemical properties, of the interaction of limonene, ethanol and Carbopol Ultrez® 10NF with the NLC dispersion, suggested that the final formulation was suitable for transdermal administration. Additionally, this formulation was not irritant.

As a proof-of-concept of the above findings, an *in vivo* transdermal administration to rats was conducted. This resulted in steady-state levels attained after 10 h and maintained for 48 h. The *in vivo* performance of the NLC dispersions was close to that obtained with hydrogels, supporting the use of the latter in a final, more convenient, formulation. This was consistent with the *in vitro* results. Skin perforation promoted by the microneedle device only slightly increased the permeation rate. This emphasized that the formulation itself provided the main driving force for skin permeation.

Overall, these findings highlight the NLC-based formulations as promising for the development of a clinical transdermal system involving simvastatin, covering an innovative therapeutic approach.

Keywords: Co-encapsulation, nanostructured lipid carriers, simvastatin, olanzapine, transdermal drug delivery, permeation enhancement

Introduction

The main challenge in transdermal drug delivery is to overcome the barrier imposed by the stratum corneum (SC), the outermost layer of the skin. Its particular composition of laterally overlapping, quasi-columnar stacks of corneocytes embedded in an intercellular medium composed by lipid multilayers is crucial for the skin barrier function [1, 2]. This limits the number of drugs able to cross it in sufficient quantities to reach a therapeutic plasma concentration. Numerous passive and active methods or the combination of both have been used to enhance the drug skin permeation [3, 4]. Within passive methods, the combination of nanotechnology and classical approaches, such as lipid nanoparticles and chemical enhancers, respectively, has emerged as a promising strategy to improve drug permeation [5]. In turn, the active transport of nanoparticles mediated by microneedle array devices has been regarded as an appealing method to facilitate drug delivery through the skin [6, 7].

This chapter addresses the use of lipid nanoparticles as both a co-encapsulating drug carrier and a strategy for transdermal administration. The latter consists of combining these carriers with common penetration enhancers in a passive approach or, alternatively, with microneedle devices in an active pre-treatment. Simvastatin and olanzapine constituted the model drugs considered for establishing this proof-of-concept.

Olanzapine (OL) is a second-generation antipsychotic drug used for the treatment of schizophrenia, bipolar mania and associated agitation [8]. Although it is more effective than other first-line second-generation drugs, the long-term use of olanzapine has been limited by its substantial, unwanted effects on lipid metabolism that result, among others, in weight gain and development of dyslipidemia, increasing the levels of triglycerides and low-density lipoprotein cholesterol, LDL-C, and decreasing high-density lipoprotein cholesterol, HDL-C [9, 10], which, in turn, leads to an increased cardiovascular risk [11, 12]. This requires a close monitoring of patients on olanzapine treatment so that, if these adverse events arise, the maintenance of the therapy may be assessed [13]. Also, in order to mitigate some of these undesirable effects, the treatment with statins, in particular simvastatin, might be required [14, 15].

Simvastatin (SV) is a lactone prodrug that is hydrolyzed *in vivo*, in the liver and non-hepatic tissues, to the corresponding β-hydroxy acid (simvastatin acid) [16, 17]. The latter is a potent inhibitor of the 3-hydroxy-3-methylglutaryl coenzyme A reductase, an enzyme involved in the cholesterol synthesis. This inhibition is mainly responsible for reducing LDL-C levels. However, simvastatin has also been shown to reduce the levels of triglycerides and increase the levels of HDL-C. Beyond that, SV is reported as effective in the reduction of the morbidity and mortality associated to the coronary heart disease [18]. This was the rationale behind the association of simvastatin, an antidyslipidemic drug, to olanzapine.

Lipid nanoparticles (LN), comprising solid lipid nanoparticles (SLN) and nanostructured lipid carriers (NLC) are colloidal carriers (40 to 1000 nm), derived from o/w emulsions, in which the liquid lipid (oil) was replaced by biodegradable and biocompatible solid lipids (that is, lipids that are in the solid state both at room and body temperatures) or mixtures of solid and liquid lipids, respectively, stabilized by an aqueous emulsifier solution [19, 20]. The use of LN for the co-encapsulation of SV and OL arise as a promising approach to promote transdermal drug delivery. Moreover, the complementarity between the therapeutics and the advantage that clearly results in the improvement of treatment compliance, the reduction in the time of production, avoidance of stability concerns and the challenge stemming from the simultaneous incorporation of drugs with different lipophilicity within the same nanocarrier, are also attractive factors from a nanotechnological point of view.

In addition, both drugs gather properties that make them suitable candidates for transdermal delivery (Table 1).

Table 1. Physicochemical and pharmacokinetic properties of olanzapine and simvastatin

Drug	Olanzapine	Simvastatin
Molecular weight	312.433	418.566
Log P/Lipophilicity	2.8[a]	4.7[b]
Aqueous solubility	3–5 μg/mL[c]	30 μg/mL[d]
Melting point	195°C[d]	135-138°C[d]
Daily oral dose	5-10 mg/day[e]	10-40 mg/day[f]
Half-life	33 h[g]	2 h[h]
Bioavailability	60%[g]	5%[h]

[a] Ref. [21], [b] Ref.[22], [c] Ref. [23], [d] Ref. [24], [e] Ref. [25], [f] Ref. [26], [g] Ref. [27], [h] Ref. [28].

SLN and NLC as colloidal systems claim several advantages for improving penetration of drugs through the skin. These include their chemical similarity to skin lipids, stemming from the common hydrophobic character, the existence of a solid matrix, and the biocompatibility, which makes these carriers suitable for long-term controlled-release skin administration. Moreover, as a result of the small particle size, a high specific surface area for drug absorption through the skin is made available, thus providing a larger efficacy as a delivery system [29]. Additionally, the adhesion of lipid nanoparticles to the skin leads to the formation of an occlusive film, causing a hydration effect associated to the reduction in transepidermal water loss [30, 31]. The resulting occlusion of the SC could also lead to a reduction of corneocyte packing and a widening of the inter-corneocyte gaps, hence facilitating drug penetration into deeper skin strata [31-33].

In turn, the use of chemical penetration enhancers (CPE) has long been shown to increase the diffusivity and/or the solubility of the drugs by reversibly disordering or 'fluidizing' the lipid structure of the SC, thus reducing the barrier resistance of the skin, among other mechanisms [3, 34, 35]. Bearing this in mind, a formulation based on CPE and lipid nanoparticles arises as an interesting approach, so as to maximize permeation, by combining the occlusive and adhesive properties of the latter with the skin permeability modifications promoted by the chemical enhancers.

A further alternative that was evaluated consists on the punctuation of the SC by a microneedle roller device (Dermaroller®). Microneedles can, in general, transiently create micropathways that allow lipid nanoparticles and drugs to bypass the SC, thus expecting a facilitated permeation into the viable epidermis [3, 36].

Preparation and Characterization of Co-Encapsulating LN: Particles with a Single Lipid

In what follows, the development of a transdermal delivery system for the simultaneous administration of simvastatin and olanzapine is described. The design of a formulation based on tripalmitin-polyvinyl alcohol SLN prepared by a modified solvent emulsification-evaporation method for SV encapsulation was the starting point [37]. Since skin hydration and the occlusion effect depend on the small size of lipid nanoparticles, an investigation about the role of different critical factors affecting the size of SLN was firstly performed. A double factorial design analysis was used so as to cover a wide range of sizes, highlighting zones with different behavior with respect to alterations in the controlled variables: lipid concentration, solvent:lipid ratio and emulsifier concentration. According to the results, the solvent:lipid ratio represented the main factor influencing particle size, and did not seem to depend on lipid or surfactant molecule. The amount of emulsifier had a non-trivial impact upon size, depending on whether systems were located below, above or close to the optimal surface coverage and, finally, the amount of lipid had a limited influence upon particle size. This analysis clearly showed that the composition parameters present a crucial role in determining the particle size of the SLN prepared by the emulsification-solvent evaporation method developed, and also facilitated the interpretation of the underlying physicochemical phenomena. The results were supported by complementary analyses obtained from differential scanning calorimetry (DSC) and attenuated total reflectance infrared (ATR-FTIR) techniques, which provided some insight into the molecular structure and arrangements, compatible with observations extracted from the experimental design. In turn, microscopy techniques allowed direct visualization of particle size and morphology, corroborating size measurements by dynamic light scattering (DLS) and laser diffractometry (LD). Finally, the SV loading only promoted minor changes upon the SLN properties [37].

Two Lipids Are Needed

However, the reduced solubility of olanzapine in the solid lipid, tripalmitin (<12 mg/g), prompted the development of NLC, based on the inclusion of an oil in the solid lipid matrix. It should be emphasized that the solubility of the drug in the melted lipid is an important precondition to ensure a sufficient entrapment efficiency [38]. Thus, in order to maximize OL loading, preliminary screening solubility studies were performed for the selection of the appropriate liquid lipid (oil). The selection included medium chain (C8-C10) triglycerides (Miglyol® 812,), polyalcohol esters of fatty acids (Labrafac® PG), and a long chain fatty acid (oleic acid) [5]. The results indicated oleic acid as the liquid lipid to be included in the formulation, not only because it allowed maximal solubility for both drugs, but also due to its enhancement permeation properties [35].

What Method for Preparing the Nanoparticles?

NLC were then prepared by two different methods: solvent emulsification-evaporation (SE/E) and high pressure homogenization (HPH) [39]. The production of NLC by SE/E was based on the previously optimized method for the preparation of SLN [40]. Briefly, both drugs, SV and OL added to the solid and liquid lipids, tripalmitin and oleic acid (50:50 weight ratio), respectively, were dissolved in dichloromethane and then added dropwise to an external aqueous phase PVA solution, under ultrasonication (40 W, 5 min; Branson, Sonifier 250). The obtained pre-dispersion was submitted to high shear homogenization (L5M-A, Silverson, UK), at 13,000 rpm for 7 min. Finally, the solvent was evaporated under magnetic stirring. On the other hand, according to the hot high pressure homogenization (HPH) technique [5], the melted lipid phase at 80°C, containing the drugs, was pre-emulsified in a polysorbate 80 solution (also at 80 ºC), using an Ultra-Turrax X1020 (Ystral GmbH, Dottingen, Germany). The pre-emulsion was further subjected to hot HPH using an Emulsiflex®-C3 (Avestin Inc., Ottawa, Canada), and after a cooling process at 4ºC, NLC were obtained. The optimal conditions for NLC prepared by HPH were also established using a 2^k full factorial planning. For that, composition variables, such as liquid:solid lipid ratio and the emulsifier concentration, and the HPH time as a production parameter, were considered the most critical independent variables. Particle size was the main dependent variable, although zeta potential and entrapment efficiency have also been assessed. The coefficients obtained from the factorial analysis indicated that the main parameter directly influencing mean particle size was the liquid:solid lipid ratio, followed by the emulsifier concentration and, to a lesser extent, the HPH time. However, the effect of the latter was marked in the interaction terms, particularly when combined with lipid ratio. This emphasized the need for establishing a thorough balance between composition and production variables to obtain particles with optimal size.

Compared with the SE/E method, the Combo-NLC prepared by HPH displayed a lower mean particle size (223.±4 *vs.* 149±18 nm), a higher polydispersity (0.122 *vs.* 0.271), but similar zeta potential (below -30 mV), which confers physical stability to NLC suspensions [41]. It should also be remarked that the diameter of the particles observed in the TEM and AFM images corroborated the DLS measurements. Additionally, AFM images of Combo-NLC indicated an irregular and rough surface (Figure 1).

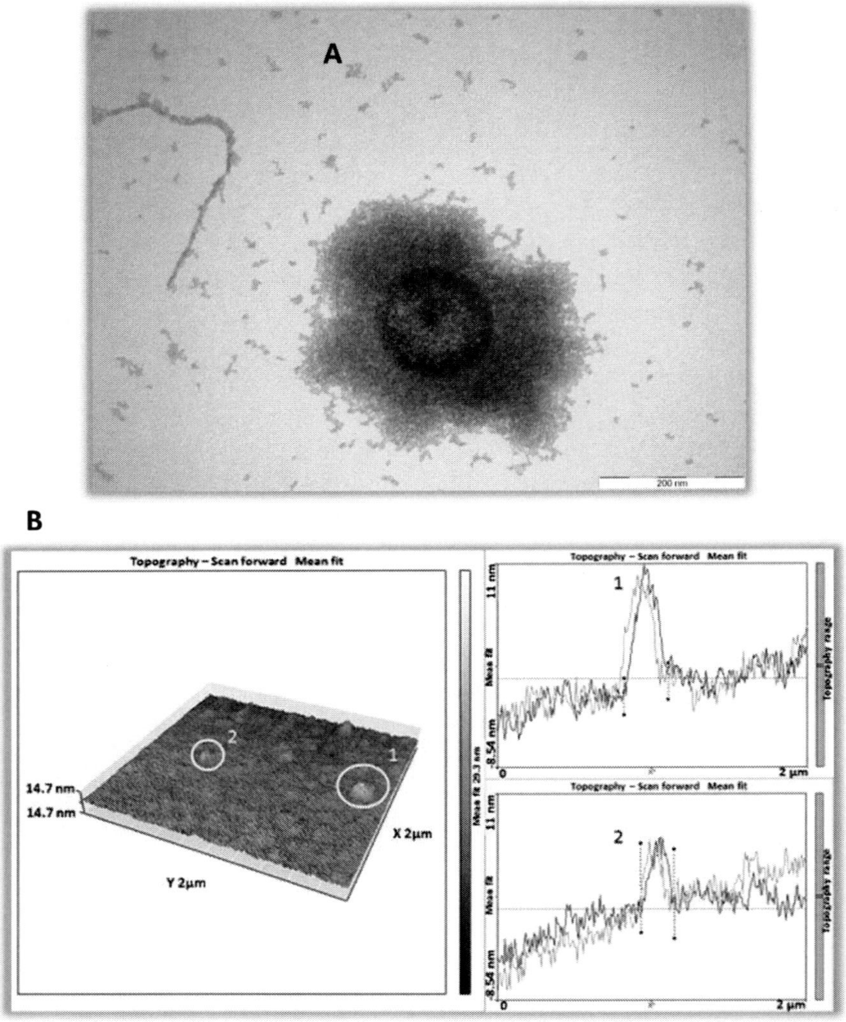

Figure 1. (A) TEM image of a particle present in the optimized Combo-NLC formulation (scale bar 200 nm) prepared by HPH, and respective (B) AFM images: 3D (left) and cross-section height profiles (right).

In addition, HPH led to an almost two-fold higher drug loading (10.637±0.005 for SV and 10.34±0.05 for OL prepared by HPH *vs.* 5.88±0.05 for SV and 5.57±0.05 in OL prepared by SE/E), associated to an entrapment efficiency exceeding 95% for both drugs, which supports the NLC as efficient carriers for co-encapsulation. These results were confirmed by DSC. The melting transition peaks of SV and OL were absent in the NLC thermograms, indicating that the drug was dissolved within the lipid matrix. A less structured matrix was associated to the NLC prepared by SE/E, evidenced by the broadness of the peak transitions and slight decrease in the enthalpy [39]. In the case of NLC prepared by HPH, the incorporation of the drugs also generally led to a decrease in the crystallinity of the lipid matrix, particularly when both drugs were entrapped. ATR-FTIR corroborated the DSC results. Spectra of NLC prepared by HPH presented several regular bands, while those obtained from NLC prepared by SE/E showed a significant convolution. The regular bands in the NLC prepared by HPH indicate a tendency for a full-trans arrangement of the methylene groups, and the mutual coupling vibrations of the long chains of tripalmitin and oleic acid [42].

Concerning the release profiles, NLC prepared by HPH tended to release drugs more slowly than those prepared by SE/E. Such a behavior was ascribed to the less structured matrix of the latter, which was in agreement with the DSC and FTIR analyses. The use of different emulsifiers, PVA in SE/E and Tween® 80 in HPH, may also have influenced results. It was observed that OL was released to a higher extent than SV, irrespective of the method of preparation. This was ascribed to their differential solubility in tripalmitin and oleic acid, which, in turn, led to different drug distribution within the NLC. SV exhibited a higher solubility in the solid lipid tripalmitin, which prompted a higher control over the release. Conversely, OL being more soluble in the liquid lipid oleic acid, the degree of retention was lower [39].

In addition, NLC prepared by HPH promoted a higher permeation rate than NLC SE/E, according to preliminary studies carried out in human skin. This was attributed to the higher drug loading obtained with HPH, despite the higher release rate observed in the SE/E formulations.

Taking into consideration the higher drug loading, the better permeation rate, and other advantages, such as the scale up feasibility, the avoidance of organic solvents and the shorter production process, NLC prepared by HPH were chosen as co-encapsulating carriers to proceed into the *in vitro/in vivo* studies.

Permeation Must Be Increased

Focusing on the transdermal co-administration of OL and SV, *in vitro* permeation studies were firstly performed using the formulation previously selected (assigned as Combo-NLC). These were carried out in static Franz diffusion cells, using newborn pig epidermis as skin model over 48 h. The preliminary parameters obtained for the Combo-NLC indicated that the degree of permeation was small. This behavior was attributed to the hydrophobic nature of the drugs that resulted in a low partition between lipid and external aqueous phase. This trend was more marked for simvastatin, the more hydrophobic drug [43].

Introducing Chemical Permeation Enhancers

A strategy to overcome this solubility related limitation consisted on the inclusion of penetration enhancers in the composition of the formulation. Ethanol, in a concentration of 30% (V/V), was firstly selected after a screening procedure involving other alcohols, such as transcutol, propylene glycol and glycofurol. The respective incorporation led to an increase in the flux at steady state of ca. 7.9 for OL and 6.4 for SV (Figure 2). Ethanol as a skin penetration enhancer promoted an alteration in the barrier properties of the skin, which was partly responsible for the high flux values obtained [44].

In an attempt to further enhance permeation, terpenes were considered to be included in the formulation. Terpenes are naturally occurring compounds derived from essential oils, which contain repeated isoprene (C_5H_8) units. Menthol (monoterpene alcohol, log P 3.23 [45]) limonene (monoterpene hydrocarbon, log P 4.58) and cineole (monoterpene ether, log P 2.82) [46] were the terpenes screened. They have been considered as very effective penetration enhancers, generally regarded as safe (GRAS) compounds in transdermal delivery [47, 48]. The terpene was dissolved in ethanol and added to the NLC dispersion in a final proportion of 30:70 (V/V). A concentration of 2% (w/V) of each one in the NLC ethanolic dispersion was firstly studied. The co-incorporation of terpenes and ethanol promoted in general a higher flux when compared to the application of ethanol alone. The tertiary combination of NLC+ethanol+limonene yielded the highest flux enhancement ratio, followed by cineole and, lastly, menthol (see Figure 2). The combined effect of ethanol and limonene has already been reported to be an effective binary enhancer system [48]. When this concentration was increased to 5% (w/V), permeation in the presence of limonene significantly augmented, yielding a flux enhancement ratio of ca. 64 and 60, respectively, for OL and SV, in relation to the Combo-NLC formulation. Conversely, in the case of menthol and cineole, an increase in the concentration led to a decrease in the permeation rate. This behavior has already been reported for menthol, having been attributed to the limited solubility of hydrophobic terpenes in 40% (V/V) of ethanol solution used in the experiments [49]. The same trend has been observed for other terpenes, although no clear explanation has been provided [50, 51].

All the above findings were corroborated by the percentage of drug permeated after 48 h, which are summarized in Figure 3.

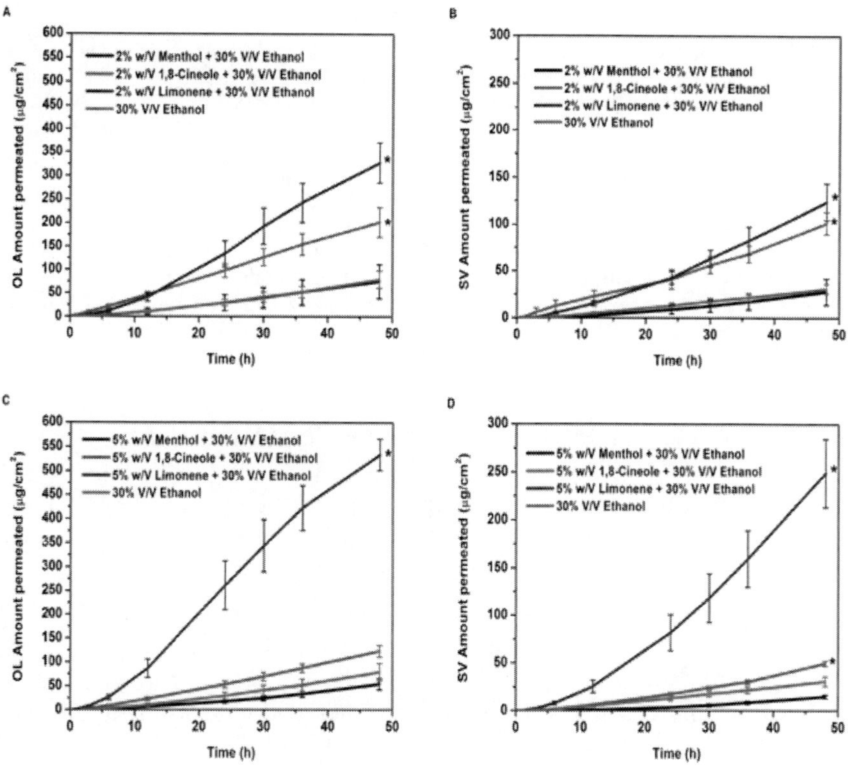

Figure 2. Olanzapine (OL) and simvastatin (SV) permeation profiles along with the different chemical (ethanol and terpenes) enhancers used in combination with Combo-NLC. * p<0.05 *vs*. 30 % ethanol dispersion as reference. b p<0.05 *vs*. NLC+30% ethanol as reference; n=3, for all the cases, with the exception of formulations NLC + 30% V/V Ethanol and NLC + 30% V/V Ethanol + 5 % w/V Limonene, for which n=6. Data are expressed as mean±SEM.

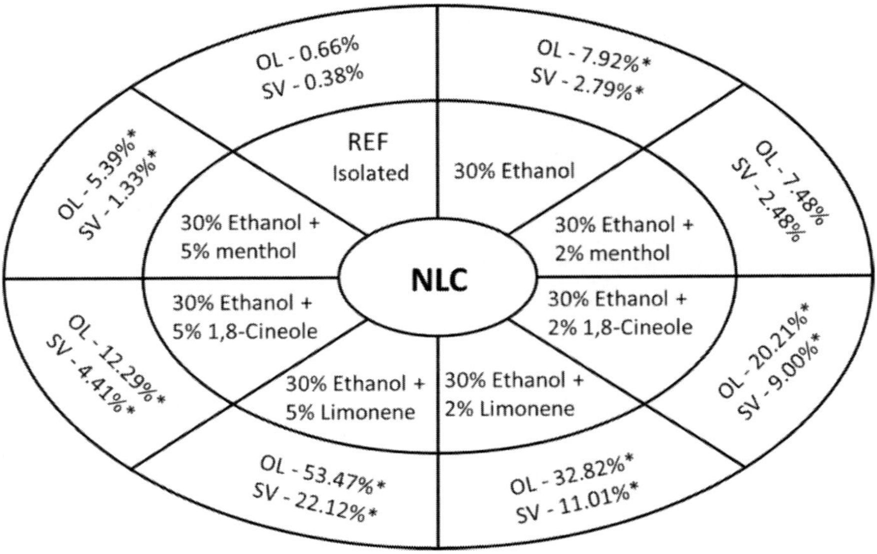

Figure 3. Different chemical (ethanol and terpenes) enhancers used in combination with Combo-NLC along with % simvastatin (SV) and olanzapine (OL) permeated after 48 h. Key: * $p<0.05$ *vs*. NLC isolated as reference (REF).

From a Molecular Perspective

To rationalize the previous results and elucidate the mechanism of action of each terpene assayed, a molecular dynamics simulation study was performed. Molecular dynamics (MD) simulations provided a route to studying the dynamics of lipid bilayers at the atomistic or near atomistic resolution, with the aim of understanding and predicting the respective macroscopic properties.

MD essentially calculates forces acting on the particles of a single input system, by solving classical Newton's equations of motion,

$$m_i \frac{\partial^2 r_i}{\partial t^2} = F_i, i = 1 \dots N'$$

with N interacting atoms, to update their positions (r) and velocities. These forces are calculated on the basis of a force field, which provides the functional form and the parameters needed for the calculation of the different potential energy terms.

MD simulations may, therefore, be used to provide insight into the interplay between the chemical penetration enhancers used and a model lipid membrane, in this case represented by dipalmitoylphosphatidylcholine (DPPC), at a level not attainable by experiment [52]. In Figure 4, the density profiles for some relevant groups of DPPC and molecules across the DPPC bilayer are depicted. These profiles showed that the limonene and cineole molecules were mostly embedded in the hydrophobic region, while menthol molecules were preferentially positioned close to the interface. Limonene was found at the interleaflet region, easily switching between the two leaflets. Menthol was, among the three terpenes under study, the one that seemed to interact more strongly with the lipid polar heads, with evidence of establishing hydrogen-bonding, and displaying a reduced probability of crossing the center of the bilayer. Representative snapshots in Figure 5, illustrate the described preferential position of each solute.

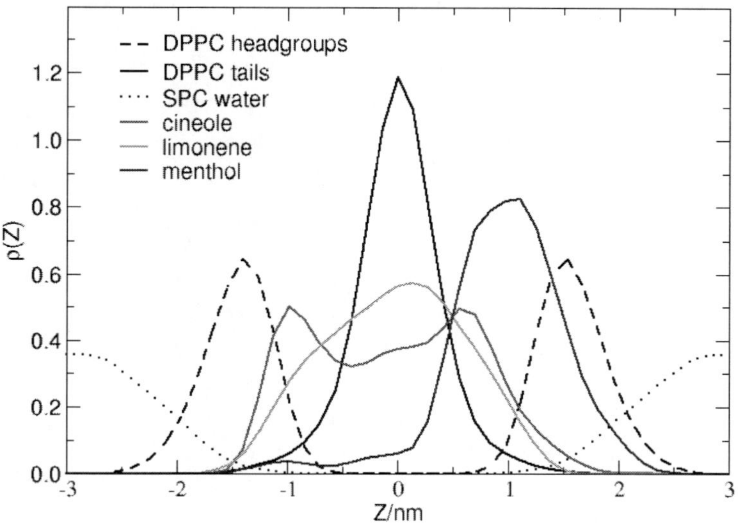

Figure 4. Probability density profiles for the terminal methyl groups of the DPPC tails (black solid line) and respective headgroups (black dashed line), SPC water (black dotted line), and for the center of mass of the inserted molecules (solid colored lines) relative to the Z-axis. Note that the Z-coordinate represents the normal to the bilayer plane and each distribution is normalized to unity.

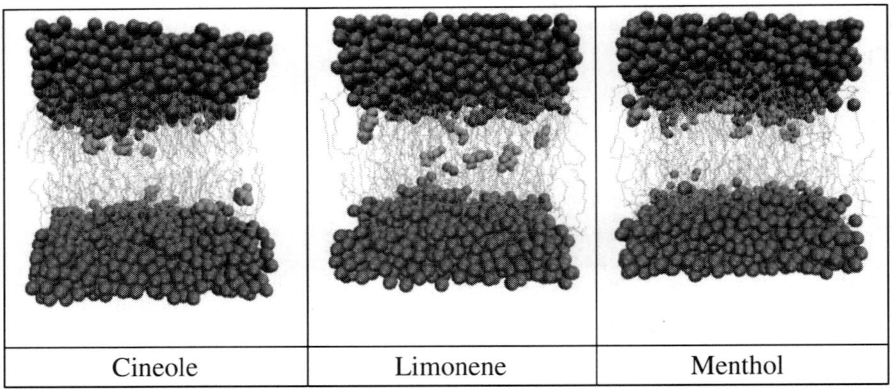

Figure 5. Snapshots illustrating typical positioning of the residues embedded in the bilayer. Key: water, terpenes and DPPC are represented in red, green and blue, respectively.

What Is Relevant and What Is Not

Based on the above findings, extracted from experimental and *in silico*/computational approaches, limonene was the terpene included in the final formulation. The next step was to quantify the permeation enhancement coming from each of the main skin penetration strategies employed, nanocarriers and chemical enhancers, represented by NLC and limonene plus ethanol as co-solvent, respectively. For that, their isolated and combined effects were assessed using a factorial planning, two-level, two-variable, 2^2, now based on permeation studies. The mathematical model applied was $R = \beta_0 + \beta_1 x_1 + \beta_2 x_2 + \beta_{12} x_1 x_2$, wherein β_0 is the arithmetic mean of the response, β_1 and β_2 are the coefficients of the respective independent variables and β_{12}, the interaction term. As independent variables, the absence (-1 level) or presence (+1 level) of limonene (5% (w/V)) and NLC were considered. A total of four different sets of experiments were carried out, in which 30% (V/V) of ethanol was always included. In the experiments without nanoparticles, saturated solutions of both drugs were prepared. As dependent or response variables, olanzapine and simvastatin fluxes at steady state, permeability coefficient, Q24 and Q48h were analysed (Table 2).

Table 2. Formulations and respective permeation parameters for simvastatin and olanzapine according to the 2^2 factorial design. Key: Et: Ethanol; L: Limonene; J_{ss} = Flux at steady-state; Kp = Permeability coefficient; Q24 and Q48 = Cumulative amount of simvastatin and olanzapine permeated after 24h and 48h, respectively; ER = Enhancement ratio. Again, the ethanol concentration is expressed in % (V/V), and that of terpenes in % (w/V). For the calculation of ER, experiment 1 was considered as reference. Data are expressed as mean±SEM. (n=6)

	Exp. #	Formulation	J_{ss} (μg/cm^2/h)	ER (J_{ss})	Kp (cm/h) (x 10^{-3})	ER (Kp)	Q24 (μg/cm^2)	Q48 (μg/cm^2)	Lag time (h)	Time* (h)
OL	1	Saturated solution (30%Et)	0.32±0.05	1.0	2.1±0.3	1.0	9.±2	15.±3	-	6.±1
	2	NLC + 30%Et	1.9±0.4	5.9	1.2±0.2	0.57	29.±7	79±18	9.±4	3.9±0.8
	3	Saturated solution (30%Et +5%L)	0.49±0.04	1.5	1.9±0.2	0.91	10.6±0.8	20.±2	-	3.5±0.8
	4	NLC + 30%Et + 5%L	15. ±2	48	10.±1	4.6	261±51	534±33	7.±5	1.3±0.3
SV	1	Saturated solution (30%Et)	0.34±0.05	1.0	1.6±0.2	1.0	8.±2	15.±3	-	7.±2
	2	NLC + 30%Et	0.74±0.08	2.2	0.42±0.05	0.26	13.±3	31.±5	10.±4	7.±2
	3	Saturated solution (30%Et + 5%L)	0.22±0.05	0.64	1.±1	0.5	7.±1	12.±2	-	7.2±0.3
	4	NLC + 30%Et + 5%L	7.0±0.8	21	3.9±0.5	2.4	82±19	249±36	14.±4	2.9±0.7

* Estimate of time after which drug is detected in the receptor compartment.

Table 3. Parameters of the response surfaces for flux at steady-state obtained from a 2^2 factorial planning in the indicated formulations and Student's t-test analysis

Response Term	β_0	β_1	β_2	β_{12}
OL J_{ss} (μg/cm^2/h)	4.498	3.395	4.093	3.307
Significance level	100.0	100.0	100.0	100.0
t value	9.059	6.836	8.242	6.660
SV J_{ss} (μg/cm^2/h)	2.077	1.537	1.797	1.598
Significance level	100.0	100.0	100.0	100.0
t value	9.665	7.150	8.361	7.437

The coefficients obtained from the factorial design stressed the higher importance of the presence of NLC in the formulation, relative to that of limonene, for the permeation enhancement, within the working ranges under consideration. This suggested that NLC acted as a drug reservoir, thus ensuring the gradient and a high driving force upon the drug, suitable for transdermal delivery, when compared with the corresponding saturated solutions. Moreover, the interaction terms indicated a synergistic action between both permeation enhancement strategies (Table 3). This was clearly illustrated by the enhancement ratio of 48 and 21, respectively for olanzapine and simvastatin, relative to the reference saturated system.

It should be remarked that the addition of limonene to the water/ethanol saturated solution promoted only a marginal increase in the flux of olanzapine, and a slight decrease in that of simvastatin. This suggested that the hydroalcoholic solution did not favor the incorporation of the enhancer into the skin. It was hypothesized that limonene was not homogeneously distributed in the solution, thus affecting particularly the partition of the most hydrophobic drug, with affinity for limonene rich domains that did not efficiently contact with the skin.

In turn, the NLC/ethanol system was a better medium to transport and incorporate limonene into the skin. It allowed a homogeneous distribution of the enhancer in the formulation, as a result of the affinity of the hydrophobic limonene to the lipid nanoparticle. Additionally, the increased contact with the skin surface determined by the small size of the particles enforces the effect of limonene, significantly increasing permeation of both drugs. It was thus shown that the external medium in the NLC dispersion had a strong influence in permeation.

Focusing now on the differential behavior of the co-encapsulated drugs, the slower permeation observed with simvastatin was again attributed to the difference in the solubility of the drugs in the lipids used as internal phase. Since simvastatin presented a higher solubility in the solid lipid, due to its solid matrix nature, the release was further sustained. In the case of olanzapine, due to its higher solubility in the liquid component, the release tended to be less controlled, thus showing a positive influence in the respective penetration degree.

Fluxes and Related Measurements

Another topic that should be remarked is related to the parameters Q24 and Q48. According to the current oral dosing regimen, a daily dose of 5 to 10 mg for olanzapine and 20 to 40 mg for simvastatin is recommended for a therapeutic effect. Since oral bioavailability is approximately 60% for OL and 5% for SV, the estimated transdermal dose should be approximately 3-6 mg and 1-2 mg per day, respectively. Thus, the target transdermal flux, according to *in vitro* permeation evaluations should be comprised between 3.1 and 6.2 μg/cm^2/h for OL, and 1.04 and 2.08 μg/cm^2/h for SV, considering a 40 cm^2 patch. This renders an amount permeated per day of 75-150 μg/cm^2 and 25-83 μg/cm^2, respectively for OL and SV. In addition, the amount permeated after 48 h (Q48) was approximately twice the amount permeated after 24 h (Q24), which suggested a constant delivery over time, even for a long-term administration. Moreover, when flux is estimated from the equation $J_{ss} = C_{ss} \times Cl/A$, taking into consideration literature values for the therapeutic blood level (Css, 0.0093 μg/mL [53] and 0.0003 μg/mL [54] for OL and SV, respectively) and clearance (Cl/F, 26100 mL/h [55] and 3749160 mL/h [54] for OL and SV, respectively, where F corresponds to the bioavailability) of typical administered oral doses of OL and SV for a specific area of skin application (A, 40 cm^2), a flow rate of 3.64 μg/cm^2/h for OL and 1.42 μg/cm^2/h for SV is obtained. Both estimates are in good agreement. The *in vitro* results obtained in the present work were above these target values and although a fine-tuning of the doses could be easily performed, it should be remarked that the results shown in this work are very promising for most common therapeutic indications.

In addition, the lag time for OL was also shorter than that of SV, and no significant difference was found for OL when limonene was added to the NLC. Although the time reported to achieve steady state for SV was increased with limonene inclusion, a higher flux with an earlier detection was obtained (see Table 2). A similar behavior was observed for OL. In turn, the reference assigned by saturated solutions did not allow the estimation of this parameter, due to the small flux evidenced. However, due to the chronic nature of these particular diseases, since the therapeutic response is ensured, the relatively long lag times were not considered an issue.

Completing the Formulation

In order to obtain viscosity values adequate for transdermal application, a hydrogel based formulation was further prepared. For that, 0.5% (w/V) of Carbopol® Ultrez 10 and the selected permeation enhancers, terpene in 30% (V/V) of ethanol, were added to the NLC dispersion, and left to hydrate under gentle magnetic agitation for 1 h. The Carbopol dispersion was subsequently neutralized using triethanolamine, so as to promote gelation. The permeation studies obtained from Combo-NLC+Et+L dispersions and the respective hydrogels, indicated a decrease in the flux (15±2 to 7.5±0.3 $\mu g/cm^2/h$ for OL and 7.0±0.8 to 3.6±0.3 $\mu g/cm^2/h$ for SV) and permeability coefficient ($10x10^{-3}$±$1x10^{-3}$ to $4.8x10^{-3}$±$0.2x10^{-3}$ cm/h for OL and $3.9x10^{-3}$±$0.5x10^{-3}$ to $2.1x10^{-3}$±$0.2x10^{-3}$ cm/h for SV) roughly by half for both drugs when the system was jellified. This behavior was attributed to the release retarding effect of the polymeric matrix and the increasing viscosity prompted by the gelling agent. Similar effects have already been reported [56]. Nevertheless, the values obtained still remained above the target flux described above, which corroborate the feasibility of transdermal delivery.

Cytotoxicity Evaluation

To investigate the potential cytotoxicity of the NLC dispersion and hydrogel formulation, the cell viability was subsequently evaluated using Df and HaCaT cell lines in a MTT assay. Firstly, the effect of the pure compounds, OL and SV, was assessed, followed by that of the NLC dispersions, including unloaded NLC, SV-NLC, OL-NLC and Combo-NLC formulations. Hydrogel formulations, with and without permeation enhancers and Combo-NLC, were also analyzed for a complete characterization. SV and OL evidenced different behaviors in terms of cell toxicity, depending on the cells tested. OL was not cytotoxic in both Df and HaCaT cells within the range of concentrations considered, 7-216 μM. SV was only cytotoxic for HaCaT cells (5-161 μM), presenting an IC50 of 12.±1 μM. This value was not significantly changed in the presence of OL (IC50 13.±1 μM). The NLC encapsulating 10 μM of SV, either alone or co-encapsulated with OL at the same concentrations, showed a cytotoxicity similar to that of the free drug, which was compatible with the release throughout the assay (Figure 6).

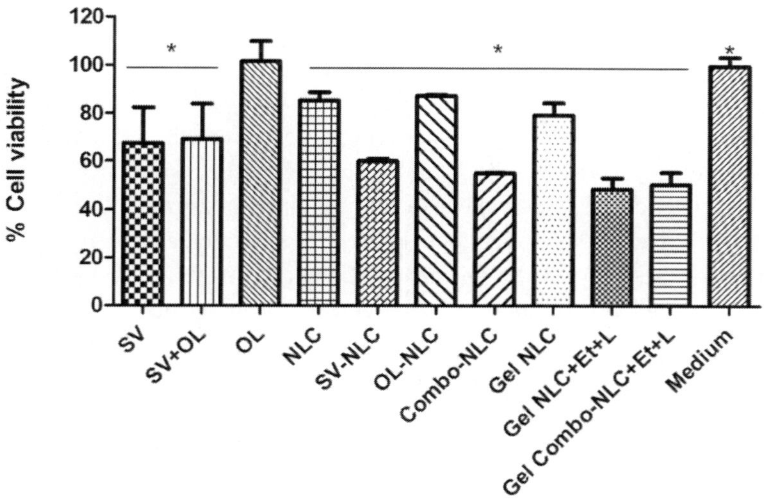

Figure 6. Viability of HaCaT cells after 72 h of incubation with SV in the concentration of 10 μM, either in the free form or incorporated into the NLC. Results pertaining to the hydrogel permeation enhancers are also presented. For these formulations, a concentration of 7 μM of SV was considered as a result of the incorporation of enhancers. Data are expressed as mean±SD. (n=9) * $p < 0.05$ *vs.* medium.

The incorporation of NLC into the hydrogel did not augment the cytotoxicity, in contrast to what happened when ethanol and limonene were added to the formulation, in which some increase was observed. However, the respective amounts are generally reported as safe and used in different applications [57, 58]. Finally, the Combo-NLC hydrogel formulation containing the permeation enhancers did not result in additional cytotoxicity. It should be remarked that, according to the relevant OECD guideline [59], an irritant substance is predicted when the mean relative tissue viability is found below 50% of the mean viability of the negative controls for a 15-60 min exposition time. In this assay, cells were exposed to test samples for 72 h with the cell viability above 50%, both for the NLC dispersion and gel. Thus, the formulations were considered non-irritant.

Size, Rheological Properties and Stability

How the different co-solvents interact with the nanoparticle formulation and contribute to the system stability and product performance were the key aspects taken subsequently into consideration from the pharmaceutical development perspective. Thus, the interaction of limonene, ethanol and Carbopol Ultrez® 10NF as gelling agent with the co-encapsulating NLC dispersion was characterized in what concerns rheological, mechanical and physicochemical properties, the latter including particle size and stability analysis. In what concerns particle size analysis, it ranged from 130 nm to 400 nm, depending on the system considered. Ethanol increased particle size, while limonene did not impact on this parameter. A swelling mechanism was proposed, corroborated by the observed increase in the steady viscosity. The inclusion of carbopol resulted in a further increase in size, which was attributed to carbomer bridging nanoparticles, resulting in some particle aggregation. However, the polydispersity index (PI) remained lower than 0.25, thus reflecting only slight differences between particle sizes within the formulation, in essentially monomodal distributions.

The rheological characterization indicated that ethanol, limonene, and NLC led to a subsequent decrease in polymer entanglement that resulted in a loss of hydrogel viscosity. Changes in the polarity of the medium and dehydration effects concurred for these observations. A more apolar medium was pointed out as a general explanation, while a polymer/nanoparticle hydrophobic interaction coupled with surfactant/polymer H-bonding provided the rationale for the NLC effect. Mechanical properties, including compressibility, hardness, adhesiveness, elasticity and cohesiveness, elucidated by the texture profile analysis confirmed the rheological findings and indicated that the optimized formulation was suitable for skin application. The inclusion of enhancers and the NLC into the hydrogel network prompted an increase in the physicochemical stability of the overall system. From a pharmaceutical and technological point of view, the results obtained allowed insight into important features that can modulate and impart formulation performance, particularly in the release and permeation behavior, as described above. Such a behavior was confirmed by ATR-FTIR spectra that revealed some disturbance order of the SC promoted by the contact with the final formulation [60].

Lastly, the inclusion of enhancers and carbomer largely contributed to the physicochemical stability of the NLC formulation, as revealed by the low transmission profiles and more negative zeta potential values. These results corroborate the findings pertaining to previous permeation and molecular dynamics simulation studies.

Active Permeation Enhancement? *In Vitro* vs. *In Vivo* Tests

As a proof-of-concept of the above findings, a pharmacokinetic study using male Sprague-Dawley rats was conducted. Rats were divided in five groups for transdermal or intravenous administrations. For transdermal administrations, four treatments were studied, based on a two-level, two-variable, 2^k full factorial planning: (1) Transdermal Combo-NLC+Et+L formulation, (2) Transdermal Combo-NLC+Et+L formulation plus skin microneedle device pre-treatment, (3) Transdermal Combo-NLC+Et+L Gel formulation, and (4) Transdermal Combo-NLC+Et+L Gel formulation plus skin microneedle pre-treatment. These groups were established taking the use of gel (x_1) and skin microneedle pre-treatment (x_2) as independent variables and pharmacokinetic parameters, such as, C_{max}, t_{max}, $AUC_{0\text{-}48h}$, C_{ss} and J_{ss} as responses (R) or dependent variables. The rats were anesthetized by isoflurane inhalation and the upper back region was carefully shaved with an electric hair clipper. The integrity of the shaved skin was checked by measuring the transepidermal water loss using a vapometer (Delfin Technology, Kuopio, Finland). A rubber ring (22 mm inner diameter and 3.5 mm thickness) delimiting a diffusion area of 3.8 cm^2 was then attached to the shaved skin with surgical glue (Vetbond®, 3M Co., St. Paul, MN, USA), in order to form a reservoir for the formulation applications. Subsequently, the transdermal formulations were applied, and the reservoir was tightly closed with Tegaderm film (3M Co., St. Paul, MN, USA), in order to prevent both formulation leakage and solvent evaporation. In the groups pretreated with microneedles, the device was rolled in four different directions, ten times for each over the rat skin surface before sticking the rubber ring. Blood samples were collected from the femoral artery catheter at predetermined time points over 48 h after formulation application and, after centrifugation the drugs were suitably extracted and quantified in the plasma [39]. On the other hand, the OL and SV solution for intravenous (IV) administration (1 mg drug per kg of body weight) was infused via the left femoral vein over 30 min, using a syringe pump (CMA 100 microdialysis pump; Phymep, Paris, France). Arterial blood samples collected over 5 h via the left femoral artery catheter were handled as described above.

What Pharmacokinetics Tells Us

The drug clearance was firstly determined through IV administration data, analyzed using a non-compartmental model, through the WinNonLin software (version 5.3, Pharsight Corporation, Mountain View, California, USA) and taking into consideration the half-life elimination time ($t_{1/2}$). The half-life of elimination from plasma was determined by linear regression of the terminal portion of the log (plasma concentration) *versus* time curves.

In the case of transdermal delivery, pharmacokinetic parameters, such as the maximal plasma drug concentration (C_{max}) and the time to reach maximal plasma concentration (t_{max}), were inspected directly from each individual plasma concentration–time profiles. The steady-state concentration of each drug was calculated by the average of the four last time points of concentration *versus* time profile, in order to calculate the transdermal flux from the dispersion/hydrogel formulation at steady state (J_{ss}) using again equation [61] $J_{ss} \times A = C_{ss} \times Cl$, where A is the area of the applied formulation, C_{ss} is the steady-state plasma concentration (ng/mL) obtained from transdermal plasma profiles and Cl the total body clearance previously determined.

The mean plasma concentration-time profiles for OL and SV after transdermal administration are depicted in Figure 7 and PK and permeation parameters are summarized in Table 4.

In general, plasma concentration reached a maximum 2 to 6 hours post skin application and then decreased to reach a plateau at around 10 h, which was maintained for 48 h (Figure 6). The C_{max} and J_{ss} values for OL were higher than those for SV, a result that was in agreement with the *in vitro* skin permeation studies previously carried out using newborn pig skin (Table 3). Microneedle pre-treatment generally resulted in earlier t_{max} and higher C_{max}. On the other hand, with the gel vehicle, the mean C_{max} values were approximately twice lower than those obtained with the liquid vehicle, while the t_{max} was delayed. This trend was confirmed by the 2^2 full factorial planning.

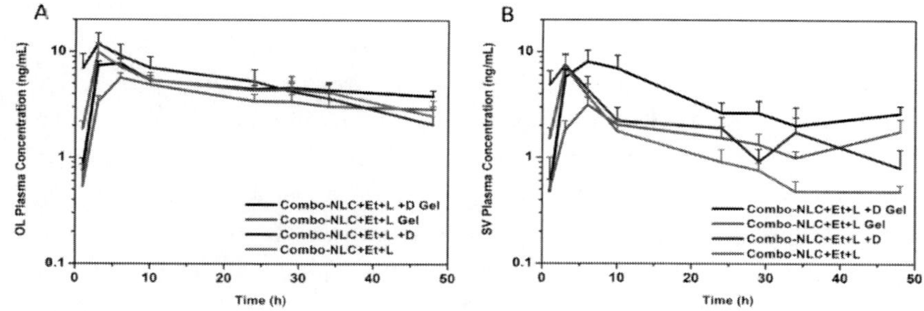

Figure 7. Plasma concentration-time curves of (a) OL and (b) SV after application of NLC plus permeation enhancers in the liquid dispersion (Combo-NLC+Et+L) or the gel (Combo-NLC+Et+L Gel) vehicle, with and without Dermaroller® (D) skin pretreatment, mean±SEM (n=6).

Table 4. Pharmacokinetic parameters of OL and SV after skin application of Combo-NLC formulations, in a liquid or gel permeation enhancer-containing vehicle. Results are expressed as mean±SD (n=6)

		Without microneedle skin pretreatment		With microneedle skin pretreatment	
Formulation		Combo-NLC+Et+L	Combo-NLC+Et+L Gel	Combo-NLC+Et+L	Combo-NLC+Et+L Gel
OL PK and skin permeation parameters	C_{max} (ng/mL)	10.1±5.2[a]	5.7±1.5	11.6±7.2	8.2±1.7[b]
	t_{max} (h)	5.0±1.6[c]	6.0±0.0	2.3±1.0	4.5±1.6[b,d]
	$AUC_{0\text{-}48}$ (ng h/mL)	214.9±99.1	171.8±66.1	220.3±172.2	229.0±52.8
	C_{ss} (ng/mL)	3.9±2.0	3.2±1.4	3.3±3.1	4.3±1.2
	J_{ss} (μg/cm2/h)	1.7±0.8	1.4±0.6	1.4±1.2	1.9±0.5
SV PK and skin permeation parameters	C_{max} (ng/mL)	7.2±5.2	3.2±1.4	8.9±4.2	8.8±5.5[b]
	t_{max} (h)	3.0±0.0	6.0±0.0	2.5±0.8	5.7±2.6[d]
	$AUC_{0\text{-}48}$ (ng h/mL)	70.0±41.2	78.0±32.5	105.8±56.8	182.3±108.[b]
	C_{ss} (ng/mL)	0.7±0.3	1.4±0.8	1.4±1.5	2.5±1.3[b]
	J_{ss} (μg/cm2/h)	0.3±0.1	0.5±0.3	0.7±0.7	0.9±0.5

Key: [a] Combo-NLC+Et+L > Combo-NLC+Et+L Gel,
[b] Combo-NLC+Et+L Gel+D > Combo-NLC+Et+L Gel,
[c] Combo-NLC+Et+L > Combo-NLC+Et+L+D,
[d] NLC+D > Gel+D, for $p<0.05$.

The *in vivo* flux for OL was 4.87 and 2.57 times higher than the corresponding to SV for NLC dispersion and hydrogel, respectively. This trend corroborated the results obtained from *in vitro* permeation fluxes. The skin perforation with the Dermaroller® produced a more marked enhancement of drug penetration and permeation for SV than for OL. The results showed that the use of a microneedle device pretreatment as an active enhancement strategy led only to a slight increase in the permeation rate of both drugs, thus indicating that the formulation itself is the more relevant factor for skin permeation. Such effect was attributed to the short lifetime of the pores created following microneedle application, which limits the clinical utility of this approach [62].

The *in vitro* fluxes were 9.18 and 5.50 times (OL) and 20.49 and 6.71 (SV) higher than the respective in vivo fluxes, for the dispersion and hydrogel formulations, respectively. The differences found was ascribed to the skin model used, rat *versus* newborn pig epidermis.

Human skin was found to be generally less permeable (about 4 times,[63]) than rat skin, but considering an increase in the application from 3.8 cm^2 to 40 cm^2, we should expect human J_{ss} values ca. 2.6 times higher than those obtained in the *in vivo* studies for the Combo-NLC gel formulation.

These values were in good agreement with previous *in vitro* estimates, thus suggesting a promising result for a possible clinical application.

Visualization

Lastly, confocal laser scanning microscopy (CLSM) was employed to visualize the distribution of Nile Red loaded-Combo-NLC within the skin, following the application of the NLC dispersion or the hydrogel formulations, with or without skin-pretreatment with 500 µm-needle Dermaroller®. Results are illustrated in Figure 8. CLSM images showed that the nanoparticles were located on upper layers of epidermis and on hair follicles and did not penetrate beyond the superficial epidermis layers. At the skin surface, Nile Red was, nevertheless, released from NLC to some extent and diffused into deeper layers, as shown by the red fluorescence of the stratum corneum (SC). The fluorescence intensity in the deeper strata was higher at 48 h than at 24 h, and was apparently more important when the hydrogel was applied. The perforation caused by the Dermaroller® pretreatment seemed to induce some damages in the SC and upper epidermis. However, after 48 h the skin seemed to have recovered, possibly due to its elastic and regenerative properties and injuries were no longer visible [62]. In summary, the NLC showed some affinity for hair follicles, and released an associated "active" into the skin.

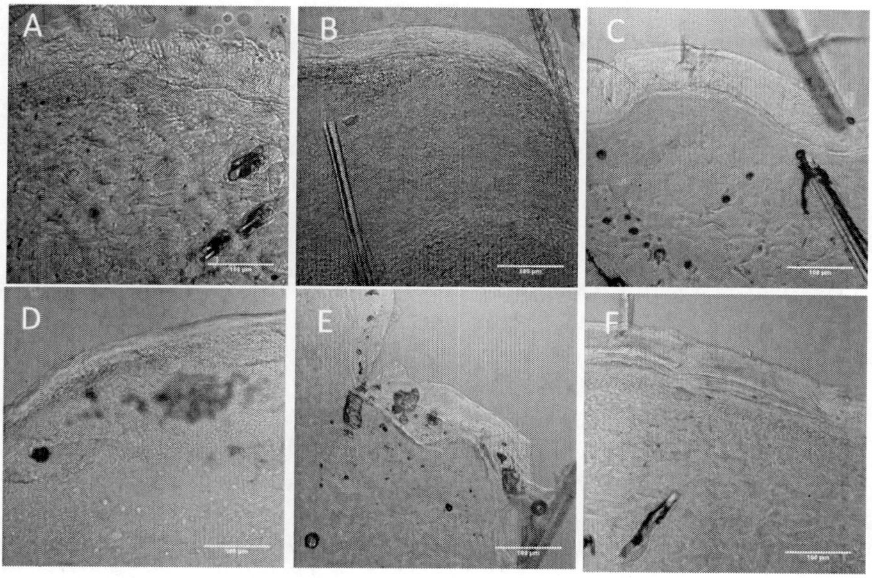

Figure 8. CLSM fluorescence micrographs revealing the penetration and distribution of the Nile Red marker within rat skin 1.5 h (a, c, e) or 48 h (b, d, f) after application of Nile-Red-loaded Combo-NLC formulation containing ethanol and limonene in the liquid (a, b) or gel (c, d, e, f) form. In (e) and (f), skin was pre-treated with 500-μm-needle Dermaroller®.

Conclusion

Lipid nanoparticles, particularly nanostructured lipid carriers, were successfully assessed as potential nanocarriers for the co-encapsulation of drugs with different lipophilicity. The development of the NLC-based formulation included optimization procedures for composition, production conditions, *in vitro* release and permeation, physicochemical characteristics, cytotoxicity, compatibility and stability analyses and, finally, *in vivo* performance.

From a technological point of view, two different methods for the preparation of the NLC were compared, namely SE/E and HPH. HPH was selected on the basis of a better performance in terms of drug loading and *in vitro* permeation rate.

Factorial designs proved to be a powerful tool for the screening procedures, and system rationalization in every development step.

In vitro versus in vivo and experimental *versus in silico* analyses of the strategies were pursued in order to strengthen the proposed mechanisms and interpretations.

The *in vitro* skin studies showed that the chemical penetration enhancers, limonene and ethanol, added to the NLC formulations, promoted a synergistic permeation enhancement of both drugs, with olanzapine exhibiting a higher permeation than simvastatin.

The *in vivo* experiments in rats correlated well with *in vitro* findings and revealed that the combined use of ethanol and limonene, incorporated in the NLC formulation provided the main driving force for drug permeation. The Dermaroller® pretreatment did not significantly enhance drug permeation, supporting the use of passive methods as suitable for a transdermal delivery system.

Furthermore, this work presented in this chapter may provide a promising proof-of-concept for further clinical application in the treatment of schizophrenia and associated disorders, combined with dyslipidemia.

References

[1] Benson HAE. Skin Structure, Function, and Permeation. Transdermal and Topical Drug Delivery: *John Wiley & Sons, Inc.*; 2011. p. 1-22.

[2] Cevc G. Lipid vesicles and other colloids as drug carriers on the skin. *Adv Drug Deliver Rev.* 2004;56(5):675-711.

[3] Alexander A, Dwivedi S, Ajazuddin, Giri TK, Saraf S, Saraf S, et al. Approaches for breaking the barriers of drug permeation through transdermal drug delivery. *J Control Release.* 2012;164(1):26-40.

[4] Barry BW. Novel mechanisms and devices to enable successful transdermal drug delivery. *Eur J Pharm Sci.* 2001;14(2):101-14.

[5] Vitorino C, Almeida J, Gonçalves LM, Almeida AJ, Sousa JJ, Pais AACC. Co-encapsulating nanostructured lipid carriers for transdermal application: From experimental design to the molecular detail. *J Control Release.* 2013;167(3):301-14.

[6] Coulman SA, Anstey A, Gateley C, Morrissey A, McLoughlin P, Allender C, et al. Microneedle mediated delivery of nanoparticles into human skin. *Int J Pharm.* 2009;366(1–2):190-200.
[7] Zhang W, Gao J, Zhu Q, Zhang M, Ding X, Wang X, et al. Penetration and distribution of PLGA nanoparticles in the human skin treated with microneedles. *Int J Pharm.* 2010;402(1–2):205-12.
[8] Kantrowitz JT, Citrome L. Olanzapine: review of safety 2008. *Expert Opin Drug Saf.* 2008;7(6):761-9.
[9] Lieberman JA, Stroup TS, McEvoy JP, Swartz MS, Rosenheck RA, Perkins DO, et al. Effectiveness of Antipsychotic Drugs in Patients with Chronic Schizophrenia. *New Engl J Med.* 2005;353(12):1209-23.
[10] McEvoy JP, Meyer JM, Goff DC, Nasrallah HA, Davis SM, Sullivan L, et al. Prevalence of the metabolic syndrome in patients with schizophrenia: Baseline results from the Clinical Antipsychotic Trials of Intervention Effectiveness (CATIE) schizophrenia trial and comparison with national estimates from NHANES III. *Schizophr Res.* 2005;80(1):19-32.
[11] Capasso RM, Lineberry TW, Bostwick JM, Decker PA, St. Sauver J. Mortality in schizophrenia and schizoaffective disorder: An Olmsted County, Minnesota cohort: 1950–2005. *Schizophr Res.* 2008;98(1):287-94.
[12] Saha S, Chant D, McGrath J. A systematic review of mortality in schizophrenia: Is the differential mortality gap worsening over time? *Arch Gen Psychiat.* 2007;64(10):1123-31.
[13] Meyer JM, Davis VG, Goff DC, McEvoy JP, Nasrallah HA, Davis SM, et al. Change in metabolic syndrome parameters with antipsychotic treatment in the CATIE Schizophrenia Trial: Prospective data from phase 1. *Schizophr Res.* 2008;101(1):273-86.
[14] Ballantyne CM, Olsson AG, Cook TJ, Mercuri MF, Pedersen TR, Kjekshus J, et al. Influence of Low High-Density Lipoprotein Cholesterol and Elevated Triglyceride on Coronary Heart Disease Events and Response to Simvastatin Therapy in 4S. *Circulation.* 2001;104(25):3046-51.
[15] Heart Protection Study Collaborative G. Effects on 11-year mortality and morbidity of lowering LDL cholesterol with simvastatin for about 5 years in 20?536 high-risk individuals: a randomised controlled trial. *The Lancet.* 2011;378(9808):2013-20.

[16] Ertürk S, Önal A, Müge Çetin S. Analytical methods for the quantitative determination of 3-hydroxy-3-methylglutaryl coenzyme A reductase inhibitors in biological samples. *J Chromatogr B.* 2003;793(2):193-205.

[17] Yang D-J, Hwang LS. Study on the conversion of three natural statins from lactone forms to their corresponding hydroxy acid forms and their determination in Pu-Erh tea. *J Chromatogr A.* 2006;1119(1–2):277-84.

[18] Kolovou GD, Vasiliadis I, Anagnostopoulou K, Cokkinos DV. Simvastatin: Two Decades in a Circle. *Cardiovasc Ther.* 2008;26(2):166-78.

[19] Müller RH, Radtke M, Wissing SA. Nanostructured lipid matrices for improved microencapsulation of drugs. *Int J Pharm.* 2002;242(1-2):121-8.

[20] Muller RH, Shegokar R, Keck CM. 20 years of lipid nanoparticles (SLN and NLC): present state of development and industrial applications. *Curr Drug Discov Technol.* 2011;8(3):207-27.

[21] Olanzapine - Compound summary, http://pubchem.ncbi.nlm.nih.gov /summary/summary.cgi?cid=4585, accessed on 16/05/2013. Available from: http://pubchem.ncbi.nlm.nih.gov/summary/summary. cgi?cid= 4585, accessed on 16/05/2013.

[22] Simvastatin - Compound Summary, http://pubchem.ncbi.nlm.nih.gov /summary/summary.cgi?cid=54454&loc=ec_rcs, accessed on 16/05/2013. Available from: http://pubchem.ncbi.nlm.nih.gov/summary /summary.cgi?cid=54454&loc=ec_rcs, accessed on 16/05/2013.

[23] Patel RB, Patel MR, Bhatt KK, Patel BG. Development and validation of an HPTLC method for determination of olanzapine in formulations. *J AOAC Int.* 2010;93(3):811-9.

[24] Moffat AC, Osselton D, Widdop B, Clarke EGC. Clarke's analysis of drugs and poisons: in pharmaceuticals, body fluids and postmortem material: *Pharmaceutical Press;* 2004.

[25] RCM Zyprexa. Available from: http://www.ema.europa.eu/docs/en_GB /document_library/EPAR_-_Product_Information/human/000115/WC500055207.pdf, accessed on 16/05/2013.

[26] Zocor RCM. Available from: http://www.infarmed.pt/infomed /download_ficheiro.php?med_id=9475&tipo_doc=rcm, accessed on 16/05/2013.

[27] Mauri MC, Volonteri LS, Colasanti A, Fiorentini A, De Gaspari IF, Bareggi SR. Clinical Pharmacokinetics of Atypical Antipsychotics: A

Critical Review of the Relationship Between Plasma Concentrations and Clinical Response. *Clin Pharmacokinet*. 2007;46(5):359-88.

[28] Schachter M. Chemical, pharmacokinetic and pharmacodynamic properties of statins: an update. *Fund Clin Pharmacol*. 2005;19(1):117-25.

[29] Muller RH, Keck CM. Challenges and solutions for the delivery of biotech drugs - a review of drug nanocrystal technology and lipid nanoparticles. *J Biotechnol*. 2004;113(1-3):151-70.

[30] Jenning V, Schäfer-Korting M, Gohla S. Vitamin A-loaded solid lipid nanoparticles for topical use: drug release properties. *J Control Release*. 2000;66(2–3):115-26.

[31] Müller RH, Petersen RD, Hommoss A, Pardeike J. Nanostructured lipid carriers (NLC) in cosmetic dermal products. *Adv Drug Deliver Rev*. 2007;59(6):522-30.

[32] Sanna V, Caria G, Mariani A. Effect of lipid nanoparticles containing fatty alcohols having different chain length on the ex vivo skin permeability of Econazole nitrate. *Powder Technol*. 2010;201(1):32-6.

[33] Puglia C, Bonina F. Lipid nanoparticles as novel delivery systems for cosmetics and dermal pharmaceuticals. Expert Opin Drug Del. 2012;9(4):429-41.

[34] Benson H. Transdermal Drug Delivery: Penetration Enhancement Techniques. *Current Drug Delivery*. 2005;2(1):23-33.

[35] Williams AC, Barry BW. Penetration enhancers. *Adv Drug Deliver Rev*. 2004;56(5):603-18.

[36] Prausnitz MR. Microneedles for transdermal drug delivery. *Adv Drug Deliver Rev*. 2004;56(5):581-7.

[37] Vitorino C, Carvalho FA, Almeida AJ, Sousa JJ, Pais AA. The size of solid lipid nanoparticles: an interpretation from experimental design. *Colloid Surface B*. 2011;84(1):117-30. Epub 2011/01/19.

[38] Subedi RK, Kang KW, Choi H-K. Preparation and characterization of solid lipid nanoparticles loaded with doxorubicin. *Eur J Pharm Sci*. 2009;37(3-4):508-13.

[39] Vitorino C, Almeida A, Sousa J, Lamarche I, Gobin P, Marchand S, et al. Passive and active strategies for transdermal delivery using co-encapsulating nanostructured lipid carriers: In vitro vs. in vivo studies. *Eur J Pharm Biopharm*. 2014;86(2):133-44.

[40] Vitorino C, Carvalho FA, Almeida AJ, Sousa JJ, Pais AACC. The size of solid lipid nanoparticles: An interpretation from experimental design. *Colloid Surface B*. 2011;84(1):117-30.

[41] Souto EB, Wissing SA, Barbosa CM, Müller RH. Evaluation of the physical stability of SLN and NLC before and after incorporation into hydrogel formulations. *Eur J Pharm Biopharm.* 2004;58(1):83-90.

[42] Lin X, Li X, Zheng L, Yu L, Zhang Q, Liu W. Preparation and characterization of monocaprate nanostructured lipid carriers. *Colloid and Surface A.* 2007;311(1-3):106-11.

[43] Walker RB, Smith EW. The role of percutaneous penetration enhancers. *Adv Drug Deliver Rev.* 1996;18(3):295-301.

[44] Narishetty STK, Panchagnula R. Transdermal delivery system for zidovudine: in vitro, ex vivo and in vivo evaluation. *Biopharm Drug Dispos.* 2004;25(1):9-20.

[45] Kang L, Yap CW, Lim PFC, Chen YZ, Ho PC, Chan YW, et al. Formulation development of transdermal dosage forms: Quantitative structure-activity relationship model for predicting activities of terpenes that enhance drug penetration through human skin. *J Control Release.* 2007;120(3):211-9.

[46] El-Kattan AF, Asbill CS, Michniak BB. The effect of terpene enhancer lipophilicity on the percutaneous permeation of hydrocortisone formulated in HPMC gel systems. *Int J Pharm.* 2000;198(2):179-89.

[47] Aqil M, Ahad A, Sultana Y, Ali A. Status of terpenes as skin penetration enhancers. Drug Discov Today. 2007;12(23–24):1061-7.

[48] Sapra B, Jain S, Tiwary A. Percutaneous Permeation Enhancement by Terpenes: Mechanistic View. *The AAPS Journal.* 2008;10(1):120-32.

[49] Kunta JR, Goskonda VR, Brotherton HO, Khan MA, Reddy IK. Effect of menthol and related terpenes on the percutaneous absorption of propranolol across excised hairless mouse skin. *J Pharm Sci.* 1997;86(12):1369-73.

[50] Kararli TT, Kirchhoff CF, Penzotti Jr SC. Enhancement of transdermal transport of azidothymidine (AZT) with novel terpene and terpene-like enhancers: *In vivo-in vitro* correlations. *J Control Release.* 1995;34(1):43-51.

[51] Nokhodchi A, Sharabiani K, Rashidi MR, Ghafourian T. The effect of terpene concentrations on the skin penetration of diclofenac sodium. *Int J Pharm.* 2007;335(1–2):97-105.

[52] Gurtovenko AA, Anwar J. Modulating the Structure and Properties of Cell Membranes: The Molecular Mechanism of Action of Dimethyl Sulfoxide. *J Phys Chem B.* 2007;111(35):10453-60.

[53] Perry PJ, Sanger T, Beasley C. Olanzapine Plasma Concentrations and Clinical Response in Acutely Ill Schizophrenic Patients. *J Clin Psychopharm.* 1997;17(6):472-7.

[54] Tubic-Grozdanis M, Hilfinger J, Amidon G, Kim J, Kijek P, Staubach P, et al. Pharmacokinetics of the CYP 3A Substrate Simvastatin following Administration of Delayed Versus Immediate Release Oral Dosage Forms. *Pharm Res.* 2008;25(7):1591-600.

[55] Callaghan JT, Bergstrom RF, Ptak LR, Beasley CM. Olanzapine: Pharmacokinetic and Pharmacodynamic Profile. *Clin Pharmacokinet.* 1999;37(3):177-93.

[56] Bhaskar K, Mohan CK, Lingam M, Mohan SJ, Venkateswarlu V, Rao YM, et al. Development of SLN and NLC Enriched Hydrogels for Transdermal Delivery of Nitrendipine: In Vitro and In Vivo Characteristics. *Drug Dev Ind Pharm.* 2009;35(1):98-113.

[57] Prasad R, Koul V, Anand S, Khar RK. Effect of DC/mDC iontophoresis and terpenes on transdermal permeation of methotrexate: In vitro study. *Int J Pharm.* 2007;333(1–2):70-8.

[58] Zhao K, Singh J. In vitro percutaneous absorption enhancement of propranolol hydrochloride through porcine epidermis by terpenes/ethanol. *J Control Release.* 1999;62(3):359-66.

[59] Test No. 439: In Vitro Skin Irritation: Reconstructed Human Epidermis Test Method. *OECD Guidelines for the Testing of Chemicals.* 2010;1(4):1-18.

[60] Vitorino C, Alves L, Antunes F, Sousa J, Pais ACC. Design of a dual nanostructured lipid carrier formulation based on physicochemical, rheological, and mechanical properties. *J Nanopart Res.* 2013;15(10):1-14.

[61] Valiveti S, Hammell DC, Paudel KS, Hamad MO, Crooks PA, Stinchcomb AL. In vivo evaluation of 3-O-alkyl ester transdermal prodrugs of naltrexone in hairless guinea pigs. *J Control Release.* 2005;102(2):509-20.

[62] Milewski M, Brogden NK, Stinchcomb AL. Current aspects of formulation efforts and pore lifetime related to microneedle treatment of skin. *Expert Opin Drug Del.* 2010;7(5):617-29.

[63] Godin B, Touitou E. Transdermal skin delivery: Predictions for humans from in vivo, ex vivo and animal models. *Adv Drug Deliver Rev.* 2007;59(11):1152-61.

In: Simvastatin Delivery
Editors: Alberto A. C. C. Pais et al.
ISBN: 978-1-63482-148-3

Chapter 4

In Situ Administration: Simvastatin in Bone Regeneration

***Susana Simões,*[1,*] *Francisco Veiga*[1], *Angel Concheiro*[2] *and Carmen Alvarez-Lorenzo*[2]**

[1] Faculty of Pharmacy and Center for Neuroscience and Cell Biology, University of Coimbra, Coimbra, Portugal

[2] Departamento de Farmacia y Tecnología Farmacéutica, Facultad de Farmacia, Universidad de Santiago de Compostela, Santiago de Compostela, Spain

Abstract

Simvastatin, a common orally administered drug for the treatment of hypercholesterolemia, has been reported to induce bone regeneration/formation and favor fracture healing. The bone anabolic effects of simvastatin are related to their ability to enhance BMP-2 expression in osteoblast cells and to reduce the formation of metabolites of the mevalonate pathway. *In vitro* studies have demonstrated that statins can increase the expression of osteogenic and angiogenic markers such as alkaline phosphatase (ALP), vascular endothelial growth factor, and

* Faculty of Pharmacy and Center for Neuroscience and Cell Biology, University of Coimbra, Coimbra, Portugal; Email: susanasimoes@ff.uc.pt.

osteocalcin in cells. Local application of simvastatin has been shown to stimulate bone formation in rodents both *in vitro* and *in vivo*. This therapeutic activity opens new ways of addressing bone pathologies (e.g., critical size defects and osteoporosis) and gives special importance to the development of new carriers to locally deliver simvastatin for the desired time periods in order to support optimal tissue regeneration *in vivo*. The potential anabolic effects of simvastatin-loaded scaffolds make them attractive candidates to support bone regeneration. Recent clinical trials show the efficacy of statins on the prevention and treatment of osteoporosis and promoting the regeneration of bone defects.

Keywords: Simvastatin, Bone regeneration, *In situ* administration, Local delivery, Clinical trials

Introduction

Search of treatments for bone deficit conditions is still a need in the 21st century medicine. Although there exist therapies that prevent/stop bone loss, few options are currently available for patients that suffer a substantial loss of skeletal bone mass. In this context, the discovery of bone anabolic agents having improved safety and promoted affordable costs is of great relevance. Simvastatin (a member of statins family) was introduced in the clinic as a cholesterol-reducing drug, but it has been also shown to increase bone mass [1-3]. Statins perform as inhibitors of 3-hydroxy-3-methylglutaryl Coenzyme A (HMG-CoA) reductase; they are able to displace the natural substrate (HMG-CoA), lowering the levels of mevalonate and subsequently the biosynthesis of cholesterol in a dose-dependent manner [2, 4]. Their hypocholesterolemic effect and usefulness in prevention of atherosclerosis rely on this mechanism [5]. Nevertheless, simultaneous inhibition of HMG-CoA reductase and disturbance of other pathways help simvastatin to cause other beneficial actions, without direct relation to cholesterol reduction. This pleiotropic effect [6] is displayed in the form of increased bone anabolism [7, 8].

The use of simvastatin and other statins for bone regeneration is a promising and growing area of research. Although the exact molecular mechanism of increase in bone formation is not entirely clear [9, 10], *in vitro* and *in vivo* evidences support the notion that stimulation of the vascular endothelial growth factor (VEGF) [11] and bone morphogenic protein-2 (BMP-2) [12, 13] due to down-regulation of prenylated small GTPase generated in the mevalonate pathway is responsible for the bone anabolic effects of statins [7, 9-11]. The increased expression of BMP-2 promotes bone formation [1, 2, 11, 12]. *In vitro* studies on induction of osteogenesis on a non-transformed osteoblast (MC3T3-E1) revealed that simvastatin activates in a dose- and time-dependent manner BMP-2 expression and subsequent increase in alkaline phosphatase activity (ALP) and mineralization [11]. Simvastatin also leads to anti-resorptive bone phenomena and inhibition of osteoclast formation [1, 2, 14-16].

Since pioneering works in 1999 [1], several treatment strategies involving simvastatin have been designed to restore bone defects. Regarding *in vivo* tests using rodents, orally administered statins have been proved to augment the bone volume in some [1, 17, 18], but not all studies [19, 20]. For example, orally administered simvastatin at 10 and 30 mg/kg/day had a negative anabolic effect on callus formation in rabbits fracture healing, whereas lower doses did not show any effect in the early stages of fracture healing [21]. Subcutaneous injection into the tissue close to the bone fracture was shown to be more effective than oral administration [1, 15]. Topical application has been demonstrated beneficial for the treatment of periodontitis, and several studies evidenced that a low dose of simvastatin is effective for recovering periodontal tissues involving alveolar bone destruction [22-26].

Local application seems to be a reasonable strategy for bone regeneration, as statins target liver metabolism and are poorly distributed to bone due to first pass elimination [27]. Furthermore, local application helps avoid systemic side effects. Thus, solid scaffolds and syringeable depots are pointed out as suitable strategies for local delivery of simvastatin in order to attain drug levels in peripheral blood circulation in the range suitable for bone anabolic effects [28-30].

From a wider perspective, *in situ* bone tissue regeneration aims to manage the biologic resources and the reparative capability of the body by means of template materials (scaffolds) that provide three-dimensional physical and biochemical support for recruitment of cells and subsequent proliferation and differentiation [31-33].

As already claimed in several studies with diverse carriers in various animal models, simvastatin may play a relevant role in *in situ* bone tissue regeneration through its regulatory effects on bone metabolism. In this chapter, the fundamentals of bone metabolism and the effects of simvastatin are revised, and then suitable doses and carriers are analyzed with the support of recent literature on *in vivo* tests. The last section is devoted to available information on performance in clinical trials.

Bone Metabolism

The intricate organization of the mineral and organic components of bone determines the mechanical performance of the skeleton [2]. Bone regeneration is controlled by complex related factors that determine formation and resorption [9] (Figure 1). Bone regeneration is compromised in a number of pathologies, and therefore there is not a single common solution for all deficiencies. In the context of regenerative medicine, the frequency and severity of bone-related illnesses make bone tissue engineering as one of the most attractive translational targets [34]. As an example, infections in bones and joints are still difficult problems with several therapeutic considerations. Critical-size bone defects resulting from traumatic injury, cancer-associated surgery or congenital malformation are still hardly addressable with available therapies [35]. Among the several challenges related to bone regeneration, achievement of adequate vascularization for the supply of cells and essential nutrients and oxygen is still a challenging task [36, 37]. Vasculature is a pre-requisite for two different processes of ossification [38]. Capillaries are required for intramembranous bone formation in order to allow mesenchymal stem cells recruitment and differentiation for the subsequent formation of bone matrix. For endochondral ossification, chondrocytes secret angiogenic growth factors that trigger proliferation of blood vessels, which in turn facilitate the access of specialized cells [39]. During bone formation, the vessels regulate the production of growth factors that determine the behavior of a variety of cells including osteoblasts and osteoclasts.

Both systemic hormones and local agents determine bone formation. The local agents are mainly growth factors (polypeptides) that directly regulate cells of osteoblastic lineage [40, 41]. In the healthy adults, remodeling of the existing skeleton is a continuous process resulting in new bone formation. This highly regulated process is sensitive to both hormonal fluctuation and aging. Although intense periods of new bone formation take place in adults during fracture healing, the matrix degradation occurring during these repairs phases causes the release of many growth factors known to be stored in bone [40, 42]. These growth factors display a critical role in the rate and extent of new bone growth [43]. Insulin-like growth factors (IGFs) or vascular endothelial growth factor (VEGF), fibroblast growth factors (FGFs), transforming growth factor b (TGF-b), and bone morphogenetic proteins (BMPs) are among the more osteoinductive agents [44]. All of these factors are incorporated into the grown matrix and presumably released in active form when bone is resorbed. The TGF family is responsible for osteoblast chemotaxis to sites of resorption defects which is required to initiate the process of formation and to stimulate proliferation of those osteoblast precursors, and is probably responsible for apoptosis of osteoclasts and cessation of the resorption phase of the remodeling process [45, 46].

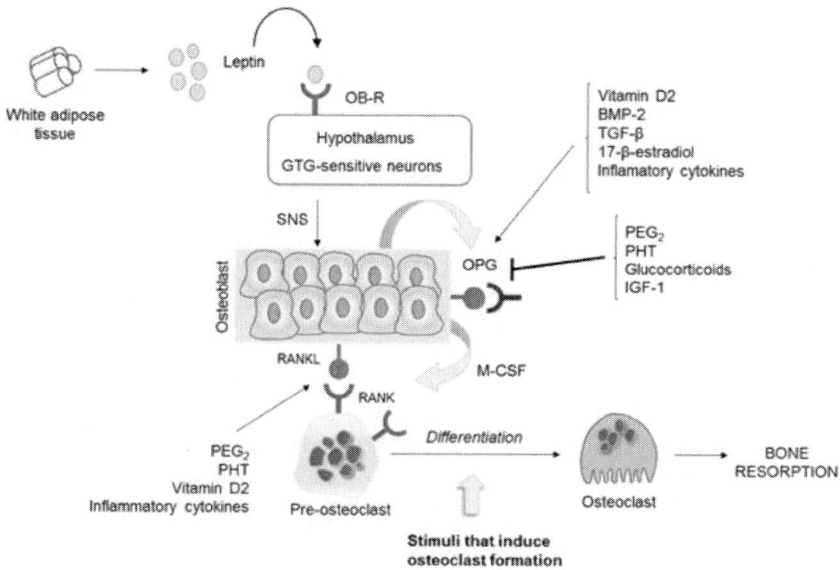

Figure 1. The role of adipose tissue and other factors in the differentiation of osteoclasts. Adapted from [56].

BMPs enhance osteoblast differentiation, including stimulation of expression of bone structural proteins such as type-1 collagen and bone matrix mineralization [47, 48]. When BMP-2 is applied *in vitro* [49] and to bone surfaces *in vivo*, there is powerful stimulation of new bone formation [50]. Recombinant BMPs, mainly rhBMP-2 and rhBMP-7, are currently approved for use in clinical applications incorporated into collagen sponges for non-union, open tibial fractures and spinal fusions [51, 52]. As an alternative, other approaches that enable minimally invasive maneuvers for implantation in the critical defect of BMP-eluting scaffolds are under study [49, 53, 54]. Nevertheless, the rapid local metabolization and the non-affordable prices of recombinant proteins are behind the search of stable osteogenic/osteoinductive synthetic molecules that resemble the biochemical stimuli to which cells are exposed in their native bone niche [49, 55].

Effect of Simvastatin on Bone Formation

In addition to the cholesterol-lowering effect, statins have a series of pleiotropic effects [57, 58]. Bone anabolism has been the focus of research for more than a decade, due to the potential clinical applications of statins to treat osteoporosis and other bone deficient processes [1, 59, 60]. Mundy and coworkers [1] discovered that simvastatin and lovastatin can stimulate high expression of BMP-2 in osteoblasts, and increase bone formation when topically applied over mice calvaria or administered orally to rats (cancellous bone volume). Subsequent studies have further confirmed that simvastatin has therapeutic action in the treatment of osteoporosis [7, 61], fracture healing [21, 58] and restoration of more bone defects [10]. The positive action of statins, mainly simvastatin, on bone formation relays on three main mechanisms: (a) osteogenesis, (b) extinction of osteoblasts apoptosis, and (c) inhibition of osteoclastogenesis [7, 10, 62, 63].

The main action of statins is the lowering of HMG-CoA reductase activity and thus of the synthesis of mevalonate. This product is an intermediate for the formation of farnesyl pyrophosphate (FPP) and geranylgeranyl pyrophosphate (GGPP), required for biosynthesis of cholesterol. Inhibition of HMG-CoA diminishes the levels of FPP and GGPP [4, 10] (Figure 2). Promotion of osteogenesis seems to be linked to mechanisms of prenylation. FPP and GGPP are required for small protein prenylation, which is needed for protein attachment to cell membranes [9, 64]. For example, prenylated Rho G has anti-osteogenic activity and promotes osteoblast differentiation [65]. Hindering the prenylation, simvastatin prevents the effects of Rho and Rho kinase. Bone formation is also favored by the increase of the expression of mRNAs encoding osteoblast differentiation markers such as BMP-2, ALP, type I collagen, bone sialoprotein (BSP) and osteocalcin [12, 13, 66]. Ayukawa and coworkers [67] found that simvastatin increases the area of bone contact with implants and the bone density, improving osseointegration.

A second mechanism deals with the ability of statins to suppress osteoblast apoptosis. Simvastatin, mevastatin and pitavastatin can inhibit up to a certain extent apoptosis, due to an increased expression of Smad3 ("mothers against decapentaplegic homolog 3") protein [68]. Smad3 proteins are signal transducers and transcriptional modulators activated by TGF-b [69]. Studies carried out in MC3T3-E1 osteoblastic cell line evidenced that the inhibition of osteoblast apoptosis is strongly dependent on the dose of simvastatin [70].

The third proposed mechanism refers to inhibition of osteoclasts and seems to be related to the impact of statins on the signaling pathway of osteoprotegerin (OPG), which is a ligand of receptor activator of nuclear factor κ B (RANK-L) and the activating nuclear factor receptor κ B (RANK). Simvastatin and mevastatin increase the expression of OPG mRNA and reduce the expression of RANKL in primary cell cultures [71, 72]. Inhibition of osteoclast function may be also favored by the up-regulating effect of simvastatin on estrogen receptor alpha (Figure 2), as observed for ovariectomized rats [73]. In addition, molecular biology and genesis reveal that both vascular and osteoblast biology have a common pathway: OPG/RANKL/RANK.

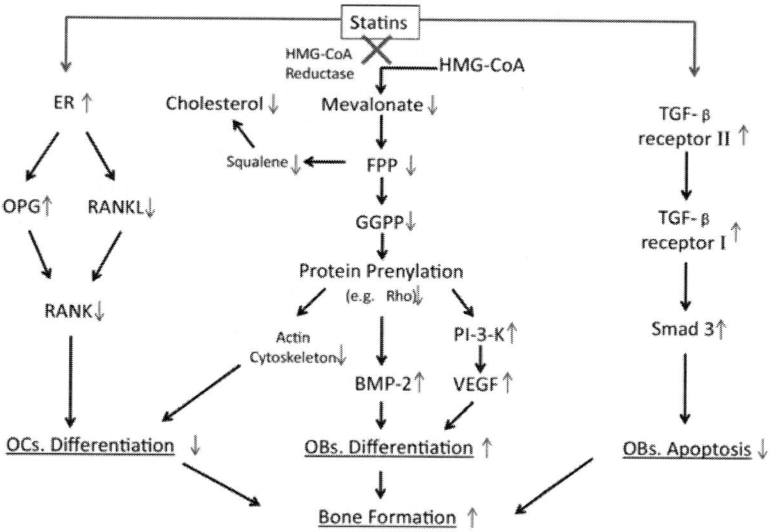

Figure 2. Pathways of statin-induced bone anabolic effects. Inhibition of mevalonate synthesis suppresses formtion of farneyl pyrophosphate (FPP) and geranylgeranyl pyrophosphatase (GGPP), which in turn stimulates BMP-2 expression and promotes osteoblasts differentiation. Statins also inhibit osteoblast apoptosis by stimulating Smad3. In addition, statins regulate the osteoprotegerin/receptor activator of nuclear factor k-B ligant/receptor activator of nuclear factor k-B (OPG/RANKL/RANK) signaling pathway by increasing the expression of estrogen receptor (ER), thereby inhibiting osteoclastogenesis. Reprinted from [10] with permission of Elsevier.

Simvastatin Local Application

Application of a bone anabolic agent at the target site or in its surroundings may markedly improve the healing of bone fractures and isolated defects (as observed in periodontitis), and facilitate the integration and stabilization of orthopedic implants. Local delivery of statins is of interest for a number of reasons. First, systemic administration can result in rare but serious side effects, most notably liver toxicity and rhabdomyolysis (inflammation of the muscle and damage) [74, 75]. Second, local administration allows an accurate dose to be placed into the desired area without depending on distribution processes and with lower risk of widespread muscle and liver damage. Additionally, the concentrations needed in the bone would be difficult to achieve through systemic delivery [76]. Nevertheless, prolonged local release is not easy and has to face up to several challenges. Small molecular weight drugs are released more quickly than large molecular weight therapeutic molecules (proteins and peptides) from scaffolds and depots, since the mesh size has less of an impact on small drugs. Thus, a precise tuning of material parameters such as hydrophilicity/hydrophobicity, swelling, crosslinking density, and rate of degradation is required [77-79]. Performance of simvastatin-loaded formulations is usually evaluated in cell cultures in terms of osteoblastic differentiation by measuring the expression of osteogenic markers such as osteocalcin, osteopontin and alkaline phosphate, and optimal effects have been shown to occur in a very narrow range of drug concentrations [60, 80]. Moreover, adequate simvastatin levels have to be combined with a scaffold endowed with osteoconductive features and suitable cell populations.

In Vitro Tests

Some studies have reported on the local delivery of simvastatin in osteoporotic bone using a biomaterial vehicle [16, 81-83]. Chou *et al.* tested beta-tricalcium phosphate (β-TCP) macrospheres for the delivery of simvastatin [82]. Drug release began to equilibrate after approximately 172 h, which can be attributed to the deposition of calcium phosphates on the material from the simulated body fluid (SBF) solution. To prolong drug release, the macrospheres were coated with apatite. The therapeutic effectiveness of β-TCP macrospheres solely and with simvastatin and of apatite-coated drug-loaded microspheres was evaluated in the right femur of osteoporotic mice and compared to the effects of the direct injection of simvastatin. Compared to the femur of the non-implanted side, all macrospheres promoted bone formation over six weeks. Mechanical analysis revealed that the stronger bones corresponded to animals treated with apatite-coated drug-loaded microspheres [82]. Similarly, Ito *et al.* introduced CaP nanocapsules [81] and CaP combined with alginate gel [83] as successful carrier materials of simvastatin in osteoporotic animal models. Bearing in mind the emerging data from osteoporotic animal models, local controlled release of simvastatin may prove as a promising approach for prevention/healing of osteoporotic fractures.

Development of injectable *in situ* gel-forming polymeric hydrogel systems has great interest in bone regeneration. Syringeable hydrogels are becoming popular as the minimally invasive maneuvers of implanting avoid relevant drawbacks of open surgery [32, 84]. Administration through a syringe allows placing the formulation into hardly accessible sites (bone defects, or tumor tissues), notably reduces the risk of infections and facilitates a prompt recovery of the patient [84-87]. As an example, Lee *et al.* reported that spaced injections of simvastatin into the mandible lead to higher bone growth (60% *vs.* 43%) and less inflammation than implantation of drug-loaded polylactic acid solid domes [88]. Park and coworkers investigated the properties of gelatin-poly(ethylene glycol)-tyramine (GPT) hydrogel as an efficient simvastatin delivery vehicle that can trigger osteogenic differentiation in the context of intervertebral disc regeneration [14]. The GPT-hydrogel system was developed using a novel enzymatic oxidative coupling reaction and display reasonable degradation and complete drug release after nearly one month in buffer containing 5% FBS. Incubation of 1 and 3 mg/mL simvastatin-loaded GTP-hydrogel with cultured MC3T3-E1 cells caused no detectable cytotoxicity yet provided a complete estrogenic differentiation for 14 days [14]. In another study, Tanigo *et al.* [86] prepared a gelatin hydrogel delivery system for simvastatin. First, simvastatin was entrapped in L-lactic acid oligomer-grafted gelatin micelles, which were then immobilized in a gelatin matrix. Simvastatin release depended on the degradation of the hydrogel, which in turn was related to the degree of crosslinking of gelatin with glutaraldehyde. Incorporation of simvastatin into the micelles led to a notable increase in apparent drug solubility and capability to induce BMP-2 production in MC3T3-E1 cells. The prolonged activity of statin-loaded micelles can be also attributed to an enhanced stability of simvastatin in the culture medium. Nevertheless, it was observed that hydrogels incorporating high amounts of simvastatin led to less bone formation. An excessive level of simvastatin may reversely suppress the BMP-2 production. Other negative effects, for example synthesis of osteosuppressive protein and induction of cell death, may happen [86].

More recently, simvastatin-loaded titanium porous surfaces were investigated regarding osteogenesis [89]. Titanium disks were pre-incubated in varying concentrations (10^{-7} mol/L to 10^{-4} mol/L) of simvastatin and preosteoblasts were directly cultured on their surface. As a control, cells were cultured on pristine titanium disks for 4, 7, and 14 days. ALP activity, type I collagen synthesis, and osteocalcin release were quantified to monitore the cellular osteoblastic activities. ALP activity increased nearly fourfold at day 4 in the presence of disks pre-soaked in simvastatin (10^{-7} mol/L) solution. Type I collagen synthesis and osteocalcin release were also maximum for the disks with a low content in drug and decreased as more simvastatin was loaded. These stimulatory effects pointed out simvastatin-bearing prosthesis as promoters of osteogenic differentiation of preosteoblasts and, as a consequence, exhibit better osseointegration [89].

Recently, block copolymers of the poloxamine (Tetronic) family have been shown able to first induce proliferation of mesenchymal stem cells, and subsequently favor differentiation to osteoblasts [49]. The unique X-shape architecture of poloxamines, with four arms of poly(ethylene oxide)-poly(propylene oxide) (PEO-PPO) blocks linked together through an ethylenediamine group, favors the self-association in the form of micelles in a certain range of concentrations at physiological pH and temperature [90, 91]. Some poloxamine varieties are cytocompatible and can form gels (with prolonged permanence in the critical bone defect) at low concentrations when combined with α-cyclodextrins (αCDs). The CDs thread onto PEO chains (forming polypseudorotaxanes) and act as reversible cross-linking points [29, 85]. Thus, an osteogenic/osteoinductive supramolecular network has been prepared combining simvastatin, poloxamine Tetronic 908 and αCDs. This gel allows solubilization and stabilization of simvastatin hydroxy acid form and synergistically promotes osteoblast differentiation [29]. The polypseudorotaxane-based gels sustained release of simvastatin for more than one week in *in vitro* tests. Proliferation and osteoblast differentiation ability of gels prepared with 4% poloxamine T908 loaded with simvastatin at 0.08 or 8.5 mM (which led to a total concentration of 0.01 and 1 mM drug in cellular medium) was compared to that of gels without simvastatin and that of conventional osteogenic medium (positive control). In various studies, both 0.01 and 1 mM simvastatin have been shown to induce osteogenic differentiation of mesenchymal stem cells, but inhibit cell proliferation [60].

(a)

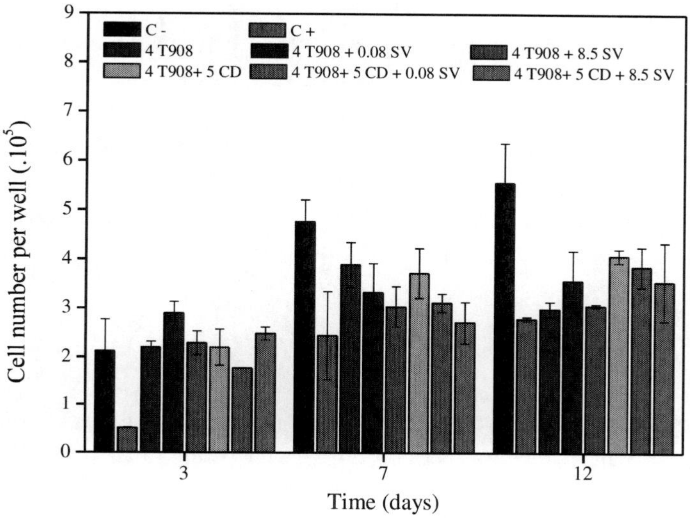

(b)

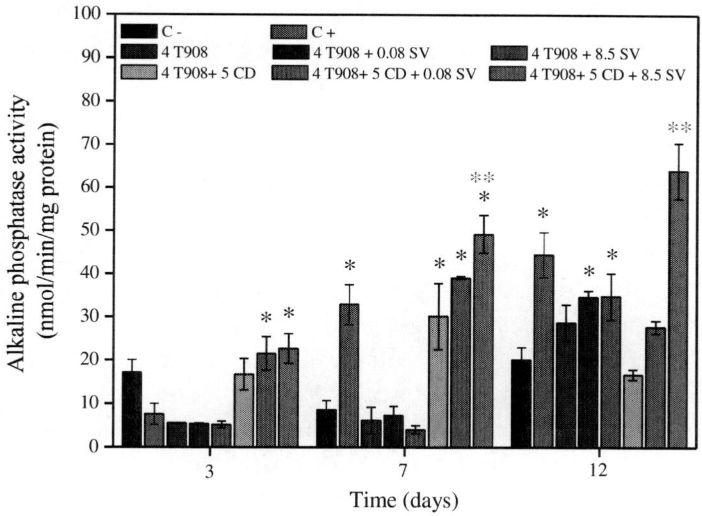

Figure 3. Viable mesenchymal stem cell number at 3, 7 and 12 days (a) and ALP activity of mesenchymal stem cells (b) in culture medium (negative control, C-), in osteogenic medium (positive control, C+) and in the presence of 4% T908 gels with and without αCD (5%) and simvastatin (0.08 and 8.5 mM). *Significantly greater than negative control ($p < 0.01$). ** Significantly greater than positive control ($p < 0.01$). Adapted from [29] with permission of WILEY-VCH Verlag GmbH & Co.

T908 gels with and without simvastatin showed proliferation levels in between those of the negative and the positive controls (Figure 3a). In the absence of αCD the osteogenic/osteoinductive effects appeared one week later than in the case of the osteogenic (positive) control medium [29]. The ALP activity was significantly larger at days 3 and 7 (ANOVA and multiple range test, $p<0.05$) for the gels containing αCD compared to poloxamine solely dispersions. Incorporation of simvastatin 8.5 mM (i.e., 1 mM in the culture medium) augmented even more the ALP activity at days 7 and 12 compared to the non-loaded gels (Figure 3b).

In Vivo Effects

Simvastatin has been reported to increase cancellous bone volume, bone formation rate and cancellous bone compressive strength *in vivo* [92]. Local application of simvastatin showed to promote fracture healing compared to control groups [15, 93]. In the first series of experiments by Mundy and coworkers the statin was injected into the subcutaneous tissue over the murine calvaria, and the effect on the underlying bone was examined [1]. There was a 30-60% increase in cortical bone width after only 5 days exposure to simvastatin and lovastatin, which was similar to the effect previously found when recombinant human BMP-2 and recombinant FGF-1 were applied in the same manner [1, 42]. Several other researchers have reported on increased bone formation in various animal models after local and systemic application of simvastatin [50, 94-96].

Skoglund *et al.* [93] systemically administered simvastatin to mice at extremely high doses of 120 mg/kg per day and observed enhanced fracture healing, although no attention was paid on any major side effects or complications derived from that exceedingly high dose. The authors concluded that additional studies with lower doses and different species are needed to establish the healing effect [93]. In another study, Chissas *et al.* [21] investigated any potential early anabolic effects of administration of low doses of simvastatin via a systemic route on a bone fracture model of male New Zealand rabbit. Two groups were orally given a diet with 10 and 30 mg/kg/day of simvastatin. The authors found a significant reduction of bone mineral density, stiffness, and energy absorbed to failure in the animals who received the highest amount of drug. Therefore, simvastatin doses of 30 mg/kg/day may have a negative anabolic effect on callus formation in rabbits, whereas doses of 10 mg/kg/day do not cause significant positive or a negative effect, especially at the early stages of fracture remodeling [21]. Differently to what happens in other species, higher doses of 50 mg/kg/day were highly toxic for rabbits, causing hepatic necrosis and death [18, 97]. These results corroborate the need of local delivery, to avoid absorption deficiencies and entero-hepatic circle, thus providing efficient drug levels in bone while overcoming the systemic collateral effects. In this regard, Wang *et al.* [15] observed that the healing process at the fractured tibiae of ovariectomised rats can be improved by means of subcutaneous injections of simvastatin (10 mg/kg/day), formulated in PBS with 2% dimethylsulfoxide and 0.1% bovine serum albumin, for a treatment period of 5 days [15].

The use of scaffolds as "*in situ*" tissue-engineered bone regeneration constructs is increasingly being investigated for local administration of simvastatin. Pişkin *et al.* [98] incorporated simvastatin into poly(ϵ-caprolactone) (PCL) electrospun scaffolds, as a novel approach to enhance osteoblastic activity and stimulate new bone formation. The fibers with or without drug were spiral-wound to generate porous 3D-matrices and then placed into cranial defects of rats for 1, 3 and 6 months. The results confirmed tissue integration and functionally stable regeneration of the calvarium in 6 months. Tissue formation was started in the macrochannels of the spiral-wound scaffolds; osteoblasts and osteoclasts migrated and proliferated from the periphery to the inner region of the matrix. The more successful bone mineralization was recorded for scaffolds prepared with simvastatin-loaded electrospun fibers, compared to scaffolds that loaded the drug via imbibition of a certain volume of simvastatin solution. The sustained release profile from the electrospun fibers resulted in an induced bone activation, resorption, and formation cycle [98].

The effect of local application of simvastatin on bone defect healing was also investigated using gelatin sponge grafts with and without simvastatin [99]. Twenty-one bone defects of 3 mm diameter were created in the angulus mandible region of Wistar albino rats. In the experimental group, nine defects were grafted with simvastatin dissolved in water mixed with a gelatin sponge. In the control groups, eight defects were filled with water mixed with a gelatin sponge alone (active control) and six were left empty (passive control) to resemble natural healing. After 14 days, the defects were prepared for radiologic and histological assessment. Density of the regenerated bone (evaluated by peripheral quantitative computed tomography) attained with the experimental group was 240% greater than that recorded for the passive control group and 190% greater than that observed for the active control group. Histologic examination also showed more new bone formation in the experimental group, leading to the conclusion that the simvastatin-loaded gelatin sponge enhanced bone defect healing in the mandible of rats [99]. In addition to sponges, gelatin hydrogels have been also shown suitable for sustained release of simvastatin *in vivo* [86]. Hydrogels incorporating simvastatin, loaded in L-lactic acid oligomers (LAo) grafted gelatin micelles, showed significant bone formation at tooth-extracted defects. Five weeks after treatment, radiographs and histological analysis showed bone regeneration of rabbit tooth defects that were treated with gelatin hydrogels incorporating 1 and 10 μg of simvastatin-LAo micelles and many osteoblasts were found in the new bone tissue (Figure 4A-D). Oppositely, little bone formation was radiographically detected in the groups treated with simvastatin in solution or non-loaded gelatin hydrogel (Figure 4A-A and B). The largest area of newly formed bone tissue was observed for the gelatin hydrogel incorporating simvastatin-LAo micelle containing 10 μg of simvastatin per site (Figure 4B-E).

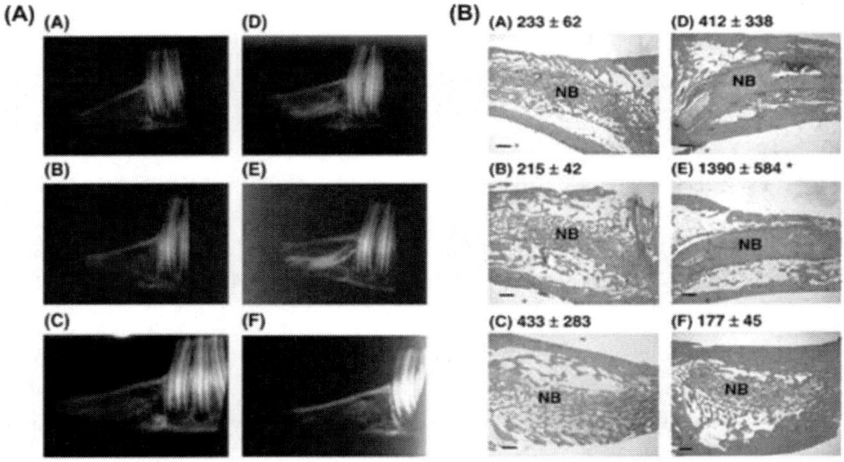

Figure 4. (A) Radiographic images and (B) histological cross-sections of rabbit tooth defects five weeks after treatment. The two series of images correspond to treatments with simvastatin solution (10 μg/site) (A), micelles-free gelatin hydrogel (B) or gelatin hydrogel containing simvastatin-loaded micelles at doses of 0 (C), 1 (D), 10 (E), and 67 μg/site (F). The molecular weight of LAo grafted and the ratio of LAo added to prepare the LAo-grafted gelatin were 1000 and 3.0, respectively. NB: newly formed bone tissue. The number indicates the area of bone tissues newly regenerated at the rabbit bone defects. *, $p < 0.05$; difference statistically significant against the bone tissue area at the tooth defect applied with other agents. Reproduced from [86] with permission of Elsevier.

Other authors also investigated the effects of locally applied simvastatin. In these studies, the doses of simvastatin used have been variable: Thylin *et al.* [95] used 2.2 mg simvastatin in 50 μl methylcellulose gel injections over rat calvaria and found a 53% increase in the thickest point of the calvarial bone after 22 days of observation. When the simvastatin-gel was implanted under a polylactide membrane, they found a 159-172% increase in bone thickness and a 144-180% increase in bone area [95]. However, the use of higher doses of simvastatin may induce inflammation, oedema, and crust formation [95, 100] and in some cases impair bone healing [100]. Wong and Rabie [101] used 0.5 mg of simvastatin in an aqueous solution mixed with collagen matrix in calvarial defects in rabbits and found a 308% increase in bone formation in grafted group relative to controls after 14 days [101]. Other good results have been obtained placing only 250 μg of simvastatin in the fracture site [59]. In this study performed by Fukui *et al.* in a mice model, non-union fractures persistent for 8 weeks were treated with gelatin hydrogels releasing a low dose of simvastatin [59]. The results showed a significant improvement in fracture healing, with 71% of the treatment group showing union, in comparison to the 7% of the control group receiving hydrogel alone. Overall, the reported findings call the attention on the relevance of designing constructs that can precisely control simvastatin release to provide appropriate drug levels.

Clinical Studies

Some authors have looked retrospectively at the abundant information available on the clinical use of statins to determine whether there is evidence supporting their effects on human skeleton. As observed in cell cultures and in animal models, statins are expected to promote bone formation in human beings via the osteoblast transcription of BMP-2 [102]. Some reports also suggest the favorable action of certain statins on prevention and treatment of osteoporosis. Several case-control studies have revealed that simvastatin administration is associated with a lowered risk of fracture [103-105], and other studies have suggested that bone mass is higher among individuals prescribed statin medications [92, 106]. However, a reanalysis of one of the previously published case-control studies [107] and another large prospective cohort study failed to find any association between statin use and fracture [105]. Post-hoc analysis from two clinical trials designed to assess the cardiovascular effects of statins found no protective effect [61, 97]. A large study involving 1375 women showed that the use of statins reduces 60% the probability of bone fracture, although this beneficial effect could not be explained only by the slight rise in bone mineral density [108]. Similar findings were recorded in men [109]. The preventive action seems to be more relevant for individuals in their 50s and older [103, 110]. In patients with type 2 diabetes mellitus, HMG-CoA reductase inhibitors have been shown to enhance bone mineral density in femur [111]. A recent prospective one year study found simvastatin treatment significant increases ALP with no significant lowering effect on bone resorption markers, which leads to enhanced bone mineral density at 6 and 12 months in women. Another study indicated an increase in serum osteocalcin levels [112]. Uzzan *et al.* [61] reported an interesting meta-analysis of 21 clinical studies, which included 3507 patients. The statins significantly increase the bone mineral density in various sites. In particular, a better effect on bone density was found by the application of lipophylic statins (simvastatin and lovastatin), which appear to be the most adequate for management of osteoporosis [61]. A recent clinical study was aimed at elucidating the effects of simvastatin and atorvastatin on bone mass and 25-hydroxyvitamin D (25OHD) level in serum [113]. A total of 114 participants having hypercholesterolemia were evaluated; 57 participants were taken simvastatin or atorvastatin (the study group) and the others did not take statins (the control group). Simvastatin and atorvastatin, at doses of 10-60 mg/day for one year, had no effect on 25OHD level but enhanced the mineral density at the lumbar spine and femoral neck [113]. Despite these positive evidences, systemic (oral) administration seems not to be an ideal method of delivery, due to the relatively low bioavailability at the fracture side and thus limited effect on bone metabolism [107, 114, 115].

There is still a paucity of information regarding local, direct application of simvastatin in bone defects in humans. The information available mainly refers to treatment of chronic periodontitis, for which the concomitant anti-inflammatory and BMP-2 stimulation features of statins may be largely beneficial to reduce the depth of periodontal pocket and to favor alveolar bone regeneration [116]. In a clinical trial carried out with smokers (> 10 cigarettes/day), patients were divided in two groups after scaling and root planning: one group was subgingivally treated with a methylcellulose gel containing simvastatin 1.2% (10 μl containing 0.12 mg) placed into the periodontal pocket, while the other group received a placebo [78]. The bleeding index, the depth of the pocket and the bone fill were notably improved in the group that received the simvastatin gel after 3, 6 and 9 months of study.

Conclusion

In the recent years a large number of studies have pointed out that statins may increase BMP-2 expression and stimulate osteoblast differentiation, promoting new bone formation. All statins currently on the market have been selected for their capacity to target the liver and decrease cholesterol biosynthesis there, and therefore they are poorly distributed to bone. Contradictory results observed in clinical trials for systemically-administered simvastatin and other statins may be related to a variety of factors such as poor oral bioavailability and dose-dependent effects on bone metabolism. Local administration appears as a promising alternative for a more accurate dosing at the target place, but demands tailored scaffolds/depots able to facilitate cell recruitment and differentiation while simvastatin is slowly released. Improved knowledge on statins therapeutic doses for bone regeneration and suitable biocompatible carriers may open novel indications for this family of drugs, which could offer a cost-effective alternative to bone morphogenic proteins.

References

[1] Mundy, G., Garrett, R., Harris, S., Chan, J., Chen, D., Rossini, G., Boyce, B., Zhao, M., Gutierrez, G. Stimulation of bone formation *in vitro* and in rodents by statins. *Science*, 1999, 286:1946-1949.

[2] Garrett, I.R., Mundy, G. The role of statins as potential targets for bone formation. *Arthritis Res. Ther.*, 2002, 4:237-240.

[3] Park, J.B. The use of simvastatin in bone regeneration. *Med. Oral Patol. Oral Cir. Bucal*, 2009, 14:e485-e488.

[4] Jadhav, S.B., Jain, G.K. Statins and osteoporosis: new role for old drugs. *J. Pharm. Pharmacol.*, 2006, 58:3-18.

[5] Blum, A., Simsolo, C., Hasin, Y. 3-Hydroxy-3-methylglutaryl coenzyme a (HMG-CoA) reductase inhibitors (statins), atherosclerosis and coronary syndromes. *Atherosclerosis*, 2004, 175:1-5.

[6] Liao, J.K., Laufs, U. Pleiotropic effects of statins. *Annu. Rev. Pharmacol. Toxicol.*, 2005, 45:89-118.

[7] Tsartsalis, A.N., Dokos, C., Kaiafa, G.D., Tsartsalis, D.N., Kattamis, A., Hatzitolios, A.I., Savopoulos, C.G. Statins, bone formation and osteoporosis: hope or hype? *Hormones*, 2012, 11:126-139.

[8] Garrett, I.R. Anabolic agents and the bone morphogenetic protein pathway. *Curr. Top. Dev. Biol.*, 2007, 78:127-171.

[9] Ruan, F., Zheng, Q., Wang, J. Mechanisms of bone anabolism regulated by statins. *Biosci. Rep.,* 2012, 32:511-519.

[10] Zhang, Y., Bradley, A.D., Wang, D., Reinhardt, R.A. Statins, bone metabolism and treatment of bone catabolic diseases. *Pharmacol. Res.*, 2014, 88:53-61.

[11] Maeda, T., Kawane, T., Horiuchi, N. Statins augment vascular endothelial growth factor expression in osteoblastic cells via inhibition of protein prenylation. *Endocrinology*., 2003, 144:681-692.

[12] Sugiyama, M., Kodama, T., Konishi, K., Abe, K., Asami, S., Oikawa, S. Compactin and simvastatin, but not pravastatin, induce bone morphogenetic protein-2 in human osteosarcoma cells. *Biochem. Biophys. Res. Commun.*, 2000, 271:688-692.

[13] Maeda, T., Matsunuma, A., Kurahashi, I., Yanagawa, T., Yoshida, H., Horiuchi, N. Induction of osteoblast differentiation indices by statins in MC3T3-E1 cells. *J. Cell. Biochem.*, 2004, 92:458-471.

[14] Park, Y., David, A., Park, K., Lin, C.-Y., Than, K., Lee, K., Park, J., Jo, I., Park, K., Yang, V. Controlled release of simvastatin from *in situ* forming hydrogel triggers bone formation in MC3T3-E1 cells. *AAPS J.,* 2013, 15:367-376.

[15] Wang, J.W., Xu, S.W., Yang, D.S., Lv, R.K. Locally applied simvastatin promotes fracture healing in ovariectomized rat. *Osteoporos Int.*, 2007, 18:1641-1650.

[16] Yang, G., Song, L., Guo, C., Zhao, S., Liu, L., He, F., Bone responses to simvastatin-loaded porous implant surfaces in an ovariectomized model. *Int. J. Oral Maxillofac. Implants,* 2012, 27:369-374.

[17] von Stechow, D., Fish, S., Yahalom, D., Bab, I., Chorev, M., Müller, R., Alexander, J.M. Does simvastatin stimulate bone formation *in vivo*? *BMC Musculoskel. Dis.,* 2003, 4:8-8.

[18] Oxlund, H., Andreassen, T.T. Simvastatin treatment partially prevents ovariectomy-induced bone loss while increasing cortical bone formation. *Bone*, 2004, 34:609-618.

[19] Yao, W., Farmer, R., Cooper, R., Chmielewski, P.A., Tian, X.Y., Setterberg, R.B., Jee, W.S.S., Lundy, M.W. Simvastatin did not prevent nor restore ovariectomy-induced bone loss in adult rats. *J. Musculoskelet. Neuronal Interact.*, 2006, 6:277-283.

[20] Maritz, F.J., Conradie, M.M., Hulley, P.A., Gopal, R., Hough, S. Effect of statins on bone mineral density and bone histomorphometry in rodents. *Arterioscler Thromb. Vasc. Biol.*, 2001, 21:1636-1641.

[21] Chissas, D., Stamatopoulos, G., Verettas, D., Kazakos, K., Papalois, A., Agrogiannis, G., Papaeliou, A., Agapitos, E., Balanika, A., Papadopoulou, E., Anastopoulos, G., Ntagiopoulos, P.G., Asimakopoulos, A. Can low doses of simvastatin enhance fracture healing? An experimental study in rabbits. *Injury,* 2010, 41:687-692.

[22] Rushinek, H., Alterman, M., Laviv, A., Weiss, E.I., Friedman, M., Casap, N. Topical application of slow-release simvastatin as a bone substitute in bone defects in the rat tibia: A pilot study. *Int. J. Oral Maxillofac. Implants,* 2014, 29:e241-e246.

[23] Montero, J., Manzano, G., Albaladejo, A. The role of topical simvastatin on bone regeneration: A systematic review. *J. Clin. Exp. Dent.*, 2014, 6:e286-e290.

[24] Stein, D., Lee, Y., Schmid, M.J., Killpack, B., Genrich, M.A., Narayana, N., Marx, D.B., Cullen, D.M., Reinhardt, R.A. Local simvastatin effects on mandibular bone growth and inflammation. *J. Periodontol.,* 2005, 76:1861-1870.

[25] Seto, H., Ohba, H., Tokunaga, K., Hama, H., Horibe, M., Nagata, T. Topical administration of simvastatin recovers alveolar bone loss in rats. *J. Periodontal Res.*, 2008, 43:261-267.

[26] de Monès, E., Schlaubitz, S., Catros, S., Fricain, J.C. Statins and alveolar bone resorption: a narrative review of preclinical and clinical studies. *Oral Surg. Oral Med. Oral Pathol. Oral Radiol.*, 2015, 119:65-73.

[27] Bellosta, S., Fed, N., Bernini, F., Paoletti, R., Corsini, A. Non-lipid-related effects of statins. *Ann. Med.*, 2000, 32:164-176.

[28] Rashidi, H., Ellis, M.J., Cartmell, S.H., Chaudhuri, J.B., (2010). Simvastatin release from poly(lactide-co-glycolide) membrane scaffolds. *Polymers* 2:709-718.

[29] Simões, S.M.N., Veiga, F., Torres-Labandeira, J.J., Ribeiro, A.C.F., Concheiro, A., Alvarez-Lorenzo, C. Poloxamine-cyclodextrin-simvastatin supramolecular systems promote osteoblast differentiation of mesenchymal stem cells. *Macromol. Biosc.*, 2013, 13:723-734.

[30] Huang, X.I.N., Huang, Z., Li, W. Highly efficient release of simvastatin from simvastatin-loaded calcium sulphate scaffolds enhances segmental bone regeneration in rabbits. *Mol. Med. Rep.*, 2014, 9:2152-2158.

[31] Ko, I.K., Lee, S.J., Atala, A., Yoo, J.J. *In situ* tissue regeneration through host stem cell recruitment. *Exp. Mol. Med.*, 2013, 45:e57-e68.

[32] Ashley, A.A., Lakshmi, S.N. Injectable hydrogels for bone and cartilage repair. *Biomed. Mater.*, 2012, 7:024105.
[33] Sanz-Herrera, J.A., García-Aznar, J.M., Doblaré, M. On scaffold designing for bone regeneration: A computational multiscale approach. *Acta Biomater.*, 2009, 5:219-229.
[34] Cowan, C.M., Soo, C., Ting, K., Wu, B. Evolving concepts in bone tissue engineering. *Curr. Top. Dev. Biol.*, 2005, 66:239-285.
[35] Khojasteh, A., Behnia, H., Naghdi, N., Esmaeelinejad, M., Alikhassy, Z., Stevens, M. Effects of different growth factors and carriers on bone regeneration: a systematic review. *Oral Surg. Oral Med. Oral Pathol. Oral Radiol.*, 2013, 116:e405-e423.
[36] Nakasa, T., Ishida, O., Sunagawa, T., Nakamae, A., Yasunaga, Y., Agung, M., Ochi, M. Prefabrication of vascularized bone graft using a combination of fibroblast growth factor-2 and vascular bundle implantation into a novel interconnected porous calcium hydroxyapatite ceramic. *J. Biomed. Mater. Res. A,* 2005, 75:350-355.
[37] Kawamura, K., Yajima, H., Ohgushi, H., Tomita, Y., Kobata, Y., Shigematsu, K., Takakura, Y. Experimental study of vascularized tissue-engineered bone grafts. *Plast Reconstr. Surg.,* 2006, 117:1471-1479.
[38] Clarkin, C.E., Emery, R.J., Pitsillides, A.A., Wheeler-Jones, C.P.D. Evaluation of VEGF-mediated signaling in primary human cells reveals a paracrine action for VEGF in osteoblast-mediated crosstalk to endothelial cells. *J. Cell. Physiol.*, 2008, 214:537-544.
[39] Chung, U., Kawaguchi, H., Takato, T., Nakamura, K. Distinct osteogenic mechanisms of bones of distinct origins. *J. Orthop. Sci.*, 2004, 9:410-414.
[40] Kini, U., Nandeesh, B.N. Physiology of bone formation, remodeling, and metabolism. In: Radionuclide and Hybrid Bone Imaging. Springer Berlin Heidelberg, 2012:29-57.
[41] Haidar, Z., Hamdy, R., Tabrizian, M. Delivery of recombinant bone morphogenetic proteins for bone regeneration and repair. Part A: Current challenges in BMP delivery. *Biotechnol. Lett.*, 2009, 31:1817-1824.
[42] Mundy, G.R., Boyce, B., Hughes, D., Wright, K., Bonewald, L., Dallas, S., Harris, S., Ghosh-Choudhury, N., Chen, D., Dunstan, C., Izbicka, E., Yoneda, T. The effects of cytokines and growth factors on osteoblastic cells. *Bone*, 1995, 17:S71-S75.
[43] Lieberman, J.R., Daluiski, A., Einhorn, T.A. The role of growth factors in the repair of bone. *J. Bone Joint. Surg. Am.*, 2002, 84:1032-1044.

[44] Cheng, H., Jiang, W., Phillips, F.M., Haydon, R.C., Peng, Y., Zhou, L., Luu, H.H., An, N., Breyer, B., Vanichakarn, P., Szatkowski, J.P., Park, J.Y., He, T.C. Osteogenic activity of the fourteen types of human bone morphogenetic proteins (BMPs). *J. Bone Joint. Surg. Am.,* 2003, 85:1544-1552.

[45] Chen, G., Deng, C., Li, Y.P. TGF-β and BMP signaling in osteoblast differentiation and bone formation. *Int. J. Biol. Sci.,* 2012, 8:272-288.

[46] Heino, T.J., Hentunen, T.A. Differentiation of osteoblasts and osteocytes from mesenchymal stem cells. *Curr. Stem Cell. Res. Ther.*, 2008, 3:131-145.

[47] Wan, M., Cao, X. BMP signaling in skeletal development. *Biochem. Biophys. Res. Commun.,* 2005, 328:651-657.

[48] Guo, X., Wang, X.F. Signaling cross-talk between TGF-β/BMP and other pathways. *Cell Res.,* 2009, 19:71-88.

[49] Rey-Rico, A., Silva, M., Couceiro, J., Concheiro, A., Alvarez-Lorenzo, C. Osteogenic efficiency of in situ gelling poloxamine systems with and without bone morphogenetic protein-2. *Eur. Cell. Mater.*, 2011, 21:317-340.

[50] Rodríguez-Evora, M., Reyes, R., Alvarez-Lorenzo, C., Concheiro, A., Delgado, A., Évora, C. Bone regeneration induced by an *in situ* gel-forming poloxamine, bone morphogenetic protein-2 system. *J. Biomed. Nanotechnol.*, 2014, 10:959-969.

[51] White, A., Vaccaro, A., Hall, J., Whang, P., Friel, B., McKee, M. Clinical applications of BMP-7/OP-1 in fractures, nonunions and spinal fusion. *Int. Orthop.*, 2007, 31:735-741.

[52] McKay, W., Peckham, S., Badura, J. A comprehensive clinical review of recombinant human bone morphogenetic protein-2 (INFUSE® Bone Graft). *Int. Orthop.*, 2007, 31:729-734.

[53] Seeherman, H.J., Bouxsein, M., Kim, H., Li, R., Li, X.J., Aiolova, M., Wozney, J.M. Recombinant human bone morphogenetic protein-2 delivered in an injectable calcium phosphate paste accelerates osteotomy-site healing in a nonhuman primate model. *J. Bone Joint. Surg. Am.*, 2004, 86:1961-1972.

[54] Bessa, P.C., Casal, M., Reis, R.L. Bone morphogenetic proteins in tissue engineering: the road from laboratory to clinic, part II (BMP delivery). *J. Tissue Eng. Regen. M.*, 2008, 2:81-96.

[55] Lo, K.W.H., Ashe, K.M., Kan, H.M., Laurencin, C.T. The role of small molecules in musculoskeletal regeneration. *Regen. Med.*, 2012, 7:535-549.

[56] Savopoulos, C., Dokos, C., Kaiafa, G., Hatzitolios, A. Adipogenesis and osteoblastogenesis: trans-differentiation in the pathophysiology of bone disorders. *Hippokratia1*, 2011, 15:18-21.

[57] Mundy, G.R. Statins and their potential for osteoporosis. *Bone,* 2001, 29:495-497.

[58] Pauly, S., Luttosch, F., Morawski, M., Haas, N.P., Schmidmaier, G., Wildemann, B. Simvastatin locally applied from a biodegradable coating of osteosynthetic implants improves fracture healing comparable to BMP-2 application. *Bone,* 2009, 45:505-511.

[59] Fukui, T., Ii, M., Shoji, T., Matsumoto, T., Mifune, Y., Kawakami, Y., Akimaru, H., Kawamoto, A., Kuroda, T., Saito, T., Tabata, Y., Kuroda, R., Kurosaka, M., Asahara, T. Therapeutic effect of local administration of low-dose simvastatin-conjugated gelatin hydrogel for fracture healing. *J. Bone Miner. Res.*, 2012, 27:1118-1131.

[60] Baek, K.H., Lee, W.Y., Oh, K.W., Tae, H.J., Lee, J.M., Lee, E.J., Han, J.H., Kang, M.I., Cha, B.Y., Lee, K.W., Son, H.Y., Kang, S.K. The effect of simvastatin on the proliferation and differentiation of human bone marrow stromal cells. *J. Korean Med. Sci.*, 2005, 20:438-444.

[61] Uzzan, B., Cohen, R., Nicolas, P., Cucherat, M., Perret, G.Y. Effects of statins on bone mineral density: A meta-analysis of clinical studies. *Bone*, 2007, 40:1581-1587.

[62] Ezirganlı, Ş., Kazancıoğlu, H.O., Mihmanlı, A., Aydın, M.Ş., Sharifov, R., Alkan, A. The effect of local simvastatin application on critical size defects in the diabetic rats. *Clin. Implant Dent. Relat. Res.*, 2014, 25:969-976.

[63] Pacheco-Pantoja, E.L., Alvarez-Nemegyei, J. Statins and osteoporosis: A latent promise. *Reumatol. Clin.*, 2014, 10:201-203.

[64] Zhang, F.L., Casey, P.J. Protein prenylation: Molecular mechanisms and functional consequences. *Annu. Rev. Biochem.*, 1996, 65:241-269.

[65] Yoshikawa, H., Yoshioka, K., Nakase, T., Itoh, K. Stimulation of ectopic bone formation in response to BMP-2 by Rho kinase inhibitor: A pilot study. *Clin. Orthop. Relat. Res.*, 2009, 467:3087-3095.

[66] Schmidmaier, R., Baumann, P., Simsek, M., Dayyani, F., Emmerich, B., Meinhardt, G. The HMG-CoA reductase inhibitor simvastatin overcomes cell adhesion-mediated drug resistance in multiple myeloma by geranylgeranylation of Rho protein and activation of Rho kinase. *Blood*, 2004, 104:1825-1832.

[67] Ayukawa, Y., Okamura, A., Koyano, K. Simvastatin promotes osteogenesis around titanium implants. *Clin. Oral Implants Res.*, 2004, 15:346-350.

[68] Kaji, H., Naito, J., Inoue, Y., Sowa, H., Sugimoto, T., Chihara, K. Statin suppresses apoptosis in osteoblastic cells: role of transforming growth factor-β-Smad3 pathway. *Horm. Metab. Res.*, 2008, 40:746-751.

[69] Lagna, G., Hata, A., Hemmati-Brivanlou, A., Massague, J. Partnership between DPC4 and SMAD proteins in TGF-β signalling pathways. *Nature*, 1996, 383:832-836.

[70] Yang, Y.M., Huang, W.D., Xie, Q.M., Xu, Z.R., Zhao, Q.J., Wu, X.M., Li, F.F., Dong, X.W. Simvastatin attenuates TNF-α-induced growth inhibition and apoptosis in murine osteoblastic MC3T3-E1 cells. *Inflamm. Res.*, 2010, 59:151-157.

[71] Kaji, H., Kanatani, M., Sugimoto, T., Chihara, K. Statins modulate the levels of osteoprotegerin/receptor activator of NFκB ligand mRNA in mouse bone-cell cultures. *Horm. Metab. Res.*, 2005, 37:589-592.

[72] Ahn, K.S., Sethi, G., Chaturvedi, M.M., Aggarwal, B.B. Simvastatin, 3-hydroxy-3-methylglutaryl coenzyme A reductase inhibitor, suppresses osteoclastogenesis induced by receptor activator of nuclear factor-κB ligand through modulation of NF-κB pathway. *Int. J. Cancer*, 2008, 123:1733-1740.

[73] Li, X., Song, Q.S., Wang, J.Y., Leng, H.J., Chen, Z.Q., Liu, Z.J., Dang, G.T., Song, C.L. Simvastatin induces estrogen receptor-alpha expression in bone, restores bone loss, and decreases ERα expression and uterine wet weight in ovariectomized rats. *J. Bone Miner. Metab.*, 2011, 29:396-403.

[74] Cohen, D.E., Anania, F.A., Chalasani, N. An assessment of statin safety by hepatologists. *Am. J. Cardiol.*, 2006, 97:S77-S81.

[75] Sinzinger, H., Wolfram, R., Peskar, B.A. Muscular side effects of statins. *J. Cardiovasc. Pharmacol.*, 2002, 40:163-171.

[76] Elavarasu, S., Suthanthiran, T.K., Naveen, D. Statins: A new era in local drug delivery. *J. Pharm. Bioallied. Sci.*, 2012, 4:248-251.

[77] Shah, S.R., Werlang, C.A., Kasper, F.K., Mikos, A.G. Novel applications of statins for bone regeneration. *Natl. Sci. Rev.*, 2015, Doi: 10.1093/nsr/nwu028.

[78] Rao, N.S., Pradeep, A.R., Bajaj, P., Kumari, M., Naik, S.B. Simvastatin local drug delivery in smokers with chronic periodontitis: A randomized controlled clinical trial. *Aust. Dent. J.*, 2013, 58:156-162.

[79] Kyllönen, L., D'Este, M., Alini, M., Eglin, D. Local drug delivery for enhancing fracture healing in osteoporotic bone. *Acta Biomater.*, 2015, 11:412-434.

[80] Song, C., Guo, Z., Ma, Q., Chen, Z., Liu, Z., Jia, H., Dang, G. Simvastatin induces osteoblastic differentiation and inhibits adipocytic differentiation in mouse bone marrow stromal cells. *Biochem. Bioph. Res. Comm.*, 2003, 308:458-462.

[81] Ito, T., Takemasa, M., Makino, K., Otsuka, M. Preparation of calcium phosphate nanocapsules including simvastatin/deoxycholic acid assembly, and their therapeutic effect in osteoporosis model mice. *J. Pharm. Pharmacol.*, 2013, 65:494-502.

[82] Chou, J., Ito, T., Otsuka, M., Ben-Nissan, B., Milthorpe, B. The effectiveness of the controlled release of simvastatin from β-TCP macrosphere in the treatment of OVX mice. *J. Tissue Eng. Regen. Med.*, 2015, Doi: 10.1002/term.1784.

[83] Ito, T., Saito, M., Uchino, T., Senna, M., Iafisco, M., Prat, M., Rimondini, L., Otsuka, M. Preparation of injectable auto-forming alginate gel containing simvastatin with amorphous calcium phosphate as a controlled release medium and their therapeutic effect in osteoporosis model rat. *J. Mater. Sci: Mater. Med.*, 2012, 23:1291-1297.

[84] Simões, S.M.N., Veiga, F., Torres-Labandeira, J.J., Ribeiro, A.C.F., Concheiro, A., Alvarez-Lorenzo, C. Syringeable self-assembled cyclodextrin gels for drug delivery. *Curr. Top. Med. Chem.*, 2014, 14:494-509.

[85] Simões, S.M.N., Veiga, F., Torres-Labandeira, J.J., Ribeiro, A.C.F., Sandez-Macho, M.I., Concheiro, A., Alvarez-Lorenzo, C. Syringeable Pluronic-α-cyclodextrin supramolecular gels for sustained delivery of vancomycin. *Eur. J. Pharm. Biopharm.*, 2012, 80:103-112.

[86] Tanigo, T., Takaoka, R., Tabata, Y. Sustained release of water-insoluble simvastatin from biodegradable hydrogel augments bone regeneration. *J. Control. Release*, 2010, 143:201-206.

[87] Concheiro, A., Alvarez-Lorenzo, C. Chemically cross-linked and grafted cyclodextrin hydrogels: From nanostructures to drug-eluting medical devices. *Adv. Drug Deliver. Rev.*, 2013, 65:1188-1203.

[88] Lee, Y., Schmid, M.J., Marx, D.B., Beatty, M.W., Cullen, D.M., Collins, M.E., Reinhardt, R.A. The effect of local simvastatin delivery strategies on mandibular bone formation *in vivo*. *Biomaterials*, 2008, 29:1940-1949.

[89] Yang, F., Zhao, S.F., Zhang, F., He, F.M., Yang, G.L. Simvastatin-loaded porous implant surfaces stimulate preosteoblasts differentiation: an *in vitro* study. *Oral Surg. Oral Med. Oral Pathol. Oral Radiol. Endod.*, 2011, 111:551-556.

[90] Alvarez-Lorenzo, C., Rey-Rico, A., Sosnik, A., Taboada, P., Concheiro, A. Poloxamine-based nanomaterials for drug delivery. *Front. Biosci. Elite Ed.*, 2010, 2:424-440.

[91] Simões, S.M., Figueiras, A.R., Veiga, F., Concheiro, A., Alvarez-Lorenzo, C. Polymeric micelles for oral drug administration enabling locoregional and systemic treatments. *Expert Opin. Drug Deliv.*, 2014, 17:1-22

[92] Montagnani, A., Gonnelli, S., Cepollaro, C., Pacini, S., Campagna, M.S., Franci, M.B., Lucani, B., Gennari, C. Effect of simvastatin treatment on bone mineral density and bone turnover in hypercholesterolemic postmenopausal women: A 1-year longitudinal study. *Bone*, 2003, 32:427-433.

[93] Skoglund, B., Forslund, C., Aspenberg, P. Simvastatin improves fracture healing in mice. *J. Bone Miner. Res.*, 2002, 17:2004-2008.

[94] Jeon, J.H., Piepgrass, W.T., Lin, Y.L., Thomas, M.V., Puleo, D.A. Localized intermittent delivery of simvastatin hydroxyacid stimulates bone formation in rats. *J. Periodontol.*, 2008, 79:1457-1464.

[95] Thylin, M.R., McConnell, J.C., Schmid, M.J., Reckling, R.R., Ojha, J., Bhattacharyya, I., Marx, D.B., Reinhardt, R.A. Effects of simvastatin gels on murine calvarial bone. *J. Periodontol.*, 2002, 73:1141-1148.

[96] Ayukawa, Y., Yasukawa, E., Moriyama, Y., Ogino, Y., Wada, H., Atsuta, I., Koyano, K. Local application of statin promotes bone repair through the suppression of osteoclasts and the enhancement of osteoblasts at bone-healing sites in rats. *Oral Surg. Oral Med. Oral Pathol. Oral Radiol. Endod.*, 2009, 107:336-342.

[97] Reid, I.R., Hague, W., Emberson, J., Baker, J., Tonkin, A., Hunt, D., MacMahon, S., Sharpe, N. Effect of pravastatin on frequency of fracture in the LIPID study: Secondly analysis of a randomised controlled trial. *Lancet*, 2001, 357:509-512.

[98] Pişkin, E., İşoğlu, İ.A., Bölgen, N., Vargel, İ., Griffiths, S., Çavuşoğlu, T., Korkusuz, P., Güzel, E., Cartmell, S. *In vivo* performance of simvastatin-loaded electrospun spiral-wound polycaprolactone scaffolds in reconstruction of cranial bone defects in the rat model. *J. Biomed. Mater. Res. A*, 2009, 90:1137-1151.

[99] Özeç, I., Kiliç, E., Gümüs, C., Göze, F. Effect of local simvastatin application on mandibular defects. *J. Craniofac. Surg.*, 2007, 18:546-550.

[100] Calixto, J.C., Villaboim de Castro Lima, C.E., Frederico, L., Lima, R., Anbinder, A.L. The influence of local administration of simvastatin in calvarial bone healing in rats. *J. Craniomaxillofac. Surg.*, 2011, 39:215-220.

[101] Wong, R.W.K., Rabie, A.B.M. Statin collagen grafts used to repair defects in the parietal bone of rabbits. *Br. J. Oral Maxillofac. Surg.*, 2003, 41:244-248.

[102] Bauer, D.C. HMG-CoA reductase inhibitors and the skeleton: A comprehensive review. *Osteoporos. Int.*, 2003, 14:273-282.

[103] Meier, C.R., Schlienger, R.G., Kraenzlin, M.E., Schlegel, B., Jick, H. HMG-CoA reductase inhibitors and the risk of fractures. *JAMA*, 2000, 283:3205-3210.

[104] Wang, P.S., Solomon, D.H., Mogun, H., Avorn, J. HMG-CoA reductase inhibitors and the risk of hip fractures in elderly patients. *JAMA*, 2000, 283:3211-3216.

[105] Chan, K.A., Andrade, S.E., Boles, M., Buist, D.S.M., Chase, G.A., Donahue, J.G., Goodman, M.J., Gurwitz, J.H., LaCroix, A.Z., Platt, R. Inhibitors of hydroxymethylglutaryl-coenzyme A reductase and risk of fracture among older women. *Lancet*, 2000, 355:2185-2188.

[106] Edwards, C.J., Hart, D.J., Spector, T.D. Oral statins and increased bone-mineral density in postmenopausal women. *Lancet*, 2000, 355:2218-2219.

[107] van Staa, T., Wegman, S., de Vries, F., Leufkens, B., Cooper, C. Use of statins and risk of fractures. *JAMA*, 2001, 285:1850-1855.

[108] Pasco, J.A., Kotowicz, M.A., Henry, M.J., Sanders, K.M., Nicholson, G.C. Statin use, bone mineral density, and fracture risk: Geelong osteoporosis study. *Arch. Intern. Med.*, 2002, 162:537-540.

[109] Funkhouser, H.L., Adera, T., Adler, R.A. Effect of HMG-CoA reductase inhibitors (statins) on bone mineral density. *J. Clin. Densitom.*, 2002, 5:151-158.

[110] El-Sohemy, A. Statin drugs and the risk of fracture. *JAMA*, 2000, 284: 1921-1922.

[111] Chung, Y.S., Lee, M.D., Lee, S.K., Kim, H.M., Fitzpatrick, L.A. HMG-CoA reductase inhibitors increase BMD in type 2 diabetes mellitus patients. *J. Clin. Endocrinol. Metab.*, 2000, 85:1137-1142.

[112] Chan, M.H., Mak, T.W., Chiu, R.W., Chow, C.C., Chan, I.H., Lam, C.W. Simvastatin increases serum osteocalcin concentration in patients treated for hypercholesterolaemia. *J. Clin. Endocrinol. Metab.*, 2001, 86:4556-4556.

[113] Thabit, A., Alhifany, A., Alsheikh, R., Namnqani, S., Al-Mohammadi, A., Elmorsy, S., Qari, M., Ardawi, M. Effect of simvastatin and atorvastatin on serum vitamin D and bone mineral density in hypercholesterolemic patients: A cross-sectional study. *J. Osteoporos.*, 2014, Article ID 468397.

[114] LaCroix, A.Z., Cauley, J., Jackson, R. Does statin use reduce risk of fracture in postmenopausal women? Results from the Womens' Health Initiative Observational Study (WHI-OS). *J. Bone Miner. Res.*, 2000, 15:S155.

[115] Rejnmark, L., Buus, N.H., Vestergaard, P., Andreasen, F., Larsen, M.L., Mosekilde, L. Statins decrease bone turnover in postmenopausal women: a cross-sectional study. *Eur. J. Clin. Invest.*, 2002, 32:581-589.

[116] Pradeep, A.R., Thorat, M.S. Clinical effect of subgingivally delivered simvastatin in the treatment of patients with chronic periodontitis: A randomized clinical trial. *J. Periodontol.*, 2010, 81:214-222.

In: Simvastatin Delivery
Editors: Alberto A. C. C. Pais et al.
ISBN: 978-1-63482-148-3

Chapter 5

The Parenteral Route: Simvastatin in Cancer Treatment

***Alaadin Alayoubi*[1], *Ahmed Abu Fayyad*[2], *Turki Al Hagbani*[2] and *Sami Nazzal*[2,*]**
[1]College of Pharmacy,
University of Tennessee Health Science Center, Memphis, TN, USA
[2]College of Health and Pharmaceutical Sciences,
University of Louisiana at Monroe, Monroe, LA, USA

Abstract

Simvastatin is a statin drug that has been widely used for the management of hypercholesterolemia. Recent studies have also suggested a role of simvastatin in the treatment of malignancies. While the exact mechanism is not completely understood, the activity of simvastatin was attributed to the inhibition of cell proliferation, induction of apoptosis and repression of tumor angiogenesis. These observations suggested that simvastatin may have the potential for use as a chemo preventive agent. The anticancer effects of simvastatin, however, were mostly observed in vitro when given in solution. Higher concentrations of simvastatin are needed to exert a similar effect in vivo. One way by which higher

* Corresponding author: Department of Basic Pharmaceutical Sciences, School of Pharmacy, College of Health and Pharmaceutical Sciences, University of Louisiana at Monroe, 1800 Bienville Drive, Monroe, LA 71201, USA, Email: nazzal@ulm.edu.

concentrations could be achieved is by the intravenous and/or parenteral administration of simvastatin. Nonetheless, due to its poor aqueous solubility, alternative lipid based parenteral drug delivery systems are needed to deliver high doses of simvastatin and to maintain elevated systemic levels. In this chapter an overview of the current research on simvastatin use for cancer treatment was highlighted. This was followed by an in depth discussion of the preparation, characterization, and anticancer activity of simvastatin loaded into nanostructured lipid carriers and parenteral lipid emulsions as promising delivery systems for the parenteral administration of simvastatin.

Keywords: cancer treatment, chemoprevention, parenteral route, nanotechnology

Introduction

Statins represent a class of drugs that are widely used for the management of hypercholesterolemia. They work by inhibiting the 3-hydroxy-3-methylglutaryl-coenzyme A (HMG-CoA) reductase, an enzyme responsible for the conversion of HMG-CoA to mevalonate, the crucial step in cholesterol biosynthesis. Recent evidence has also suggested a role of statins in the treatment of malignancies [1]. In several studies, statins were shown to induce cell cycle arrest in vitro [2-5] and to inhibit breast, pancreas, liver, and prostate tumor cell growth [6-8].

The exact nature of the anti-proliferative and pro-apoptotic effects of statins on cancer cells is, however, not completely understood. The effect may be attributed to the inhibition of mevalonate synthesis, which plays an important role in geranylgeranylation and farnesylation of the Rho and Ras GTPases [9]. Rho proteins are involved in the proliferative and invasiveness of cancers [10-15]. Therefore, inhibition of geranylgeranylation of Rho may represent a potent mechanism for statin-induced attenuation of cancer cell growth.

In vivo studies have also shown that simvastatin increases transcription of phosphatase and tensin homolog (PTEN) which inhibits the oncogenic phosphatidylinositol-3-kinase (PI3K) pathway. Moreover, simvastatin was found to inhibit DNA binding of the NF-kB transcription factor which reduces the expression of several anti-apoptotic proteins [16]. NF-kB induces genes that code for antiapoptotic proteins such as cFLIP and cIAP [17, 18]. cFLIP inhibits apoptosis by binding to Fas-associated death domain protein (FADD) and procaspase-8 [19, 20]. cIAP directly binds and inhibits effector caspases, acting downstream of initiator caspases [21]. In addition, NF-kB induces expression of several Bcl-2 family members that are involved in mitochondrial-mediated apoptosis, most notably Bcl-xL, which prevents apoptosis by inhibiting permeability transition and depolarization of mitochondria and blocking cytochrome c release [35, 36]. By increasing DNA fragmentation and overexpression of pro-apoptotic gene Bax together with an inhibition of BCL-2; the gene that encodes for Bcl-2, simvastatin induces apoptosis in cancer cells without affecting the normal cells [22-24]. Furthermore, the ischemic necrosis of tumors treated with simvastatin suggests that simvastatin inhibits angiogenesis. Since VEGF, which plays a central role in angiogenesis by promoting the growth of vascular endothelial cells and enhancing vascular permeability [25], is known to be regulated by NF-kB [26-28], it is possible that simvastatin inhibits VEGF-mediated angiogenesis via the NF-kB pathway.

Based on these findings, the anticancer effects of simvastatin could be attributed not only to the inhibition of cell proliferation, but also to apoptosis and repression of tumor angiogenesis. Since evading apoptosis is one of the hallmarks of cancer [29], the induction of apoptosis by simvastatin suggests that it could be used as a chemo preventive agent. The anticancer effects of simvastatin were already observed in vitro and in vivo. However, higher concentrations of simvastatin are needed to exert an effect in vivo similar to that seen in vitro [30]. One way by which higher concentrations could be achieved is by intravenous and/or parenteral administration of statins [31].

Parenteral Administration of Simvastatin

Drugs in general are administered by either an enteral or a parenteral route of administration. Enteral route usually refers to the administration of drugs or drug products via the oral, sublingual, or rectal route, i.e., administration to the gastrointestinal tract. The term parenteral, on the other hand, is derived from the Greek words para, meaning beside, and enteron, meaning intestine, which together indicate an application outside of the intestine and not by way of the alimentary tract. The term parenteral administration, however, is often used to refer to the injection of a drug or drug product via a needle into the body at various sites and to various depths [32]. Subcutaneous, intramuscular, and intravenous administration are the primary routes of parenteral administration, although other routes such as intracardiac, intraperitoneal, and intraspinal have also been used for drug administration.

Overall, parenteral administration is preferred when rapid absorption is essential. Blood levels after parenteral administration are also more predictable than after oral administration. The parenteral route of administration is especially useful in treating patients who are uncooperative, unconscious, or otherwise unable to accept oral medication [32]. In light of these advantages, parenteral administration could be used to sustain high concentrations of simvastatin needed to elicit anticancer effects. Several studies have already been reported in the literature in which simvastatin was administered parentally for potential use in cancer therapy. An excerpt of studies in which simvastatin was reported to have been administered parenterally is summarized in Table 1. Also shown in this table are the administered dose and the observed effects in vitro and/or in vivo.

In the majority of these studies simvastatin treatment was carried out by the intraperitoneal administration of an aqueous solution or an oil dispersion. Only small doses of simvastatin however could be administered via these vehicles due to its poor aqueous solubility. The development of new injectable drug delivery systems is therefore needed to maintain high systemic drug levels. Several technologies have been developed for the parenteral delivery of poorly soluble drugs. For example, biodegradable in situ forming implants, such as Eligard® have been developed to control the release of drug substances and to obtain defined blood levels over a specified time. These implant systems are made of biodegradable products, which can be injected via a syringe into the body. Once injected, they solidify to form a semi-solid depot [33]. A similar approach was used to improve the bioavailability of simvastatin. A study was reported in which a solid implant was formed after intraperitoneal injection of a polymeric solution containing simvastatin. It sustained simvastatin release for up to 15 days with no adverse drug polymer interactions. A three-fold increase in bioavailability was also observed when compared to commercial product ZOCOR® 10 mg tablets [34]. Alternative technologies, such as nanostructured lipid carriers and nanoemulsions have also been reported for the parenteral delivery of simvastatin.

Table 1. An overview of studies in which simvastatin was parenterally administered and tested for its anticancer activity

Simvastatin dose	RA[1]	Solvent system	*In Vitro* Cell line	*In Vivo* model	Cancer type	Results	Reference
2 mg/kg every 12 h	i.p.[2]	DMEM[3]	Human PC3 and LNCaP[4]	Nude Mouse Tumor Xenograft	Prostate cancer	Long-term simvastatin medication may have beneficial effects in the management of Prostate cancer.	[35]
5 mg/kg	i.p.	Suspended in corn oil	Gastric cancer cell lines (SNU-5, SNU-16, MKN45 and AGS)	Xenograft gastric tumor mouse	Gastric cancer	Simvastatin has significant potential for the treatment of gastric cancer	[36]
5 mg/kg (+ 60 mg/Kg capecitabine)	i.p.	Suspended in corn oil	Gastric cancer cell lines (SNU-5, SNU-16, MKN45 and AGS)	Xenograft gastric tumor mouse	Gastric cancer	Simvastatin effects can be further enhanced by capecitabine for treatment of gastric cancer	[36]
5 mg/kg	Injected in the left cardiac ventricle	N/A	BT-20 human breast cancer	Nude mice	Skeletal Metastasis of Breast Cancer	Simvastatin prevents osteolytic bone metastasis of breast cancer cells by	[37]

Table 1. (Continued)

Simvastatin dose	**RA**[1]	**Solvent system**	***In Vitro* Cell line**	***In Vivo* model**	**Cancer type**	**Results**	**Reference**
						increasing the levels of mutated p53	
1 μg/g	i.p.	DMSO[5]	B16-F10 melanoma cells and two human SK-Mel-3 and A375 melanoma cells.	Murine model	Melanoma	Simvastatin induces a strong downregulation in the expression of NonO, the murine homolog of p54nrb.	[38]
2mg/kg every 12h for 2 weeks	i.p.	N/A	Human PC3 and LNCaP	Nude mouse tumor xenograft model	Prostate cancer	Treatment with simvastatin both *in vitro* and *in vivo* significantly induced apoptosis in prostate cancer cells	[39]
15-20mg/kg every day for 2 weeks	s.c.[6] infusion	Water	Murine leukemia P338D1	SCID[7]	Myeloid leukemia	Inhibition of Acute Myeloid Leukemia cell proliferation by simvastatin may be independent of the	[40]

Simvastatin dose	**RA[1]**	**Solvent system**	***In Vitro* Cell line**	***In Vivo* model**	**Cancer type**	**Results**	**Reference**
						RAS[8] signaling pathway.	
2 mg/kg (+ 10 mg/kg cetuximab)	i.p.	PBS[9]	CRC[10]	Xenograft tumor mouse	Colorectal cancer	Simvastatin may overcome cetuximab resistance in colon cancer cells with KRAS[11] mutations by modulating BRAF[12] activity and inducing apoptosis	[41]
0.2 mM (+ 2.5 mg/kg bevacizumab)	i.p.	DW[13]	11 human CRC cell lines, CoLo320, DiFi, NCI-H716, SW48, HT29, RKO, WiDr, DLD1, HCT8, LS174T, and SW403	xenograft tumors	Colorectal cancer	Simvastatin at doses used in patients with cardiovascular diseases (40–80 mg once daily) may potentiate the anti-angiogenic effects of bevacizumab on CRC by suppressing angiopoietin2, BiP, and Hsp90a in cancer cells	[42]

Table 1. (Continued)

Simvastatin dose	RA[1]	Solvent system	*In Vitro* Cell line	*In Vivo* model	Cancer type	Results	Reference
10 mg/kg	i.p.	EtOH[14] with NaOH solution	-	Genetically engineered mouse model	Pancreatic cancer	Simvastatin has potential to delay the formation of pancreatic cancer and its precursor Lesions, which support the hypothesis that statins might be a valid chemopreventive strategy in delaying PanIN[15]	[43]

ABBREVIATIONS: [1]RA: Route of Administration, [2]i.p.: Intra Peritoneal, [3]DMEM: Dulbecco's Modified Eagle Medium, [4]LNCaP: lymph node carcinoma of the prostate, [5]DMSO: Dimethyl sulfoxide, [6]s.c.: Subcutaneous, [7]SCID: Severe combined immunedeficient mice, [8]RAS: Rat sarcoma, [9]PBS: Phosphate buffered saline, [10]CRC: Human metastatic colorectal cancer, [11]KRAS: Kirsten rat sarcoma viral oncogene homolog, [12]BRAF: A human gene that makes a protein called B-Raf, [13]DW: Distilled water, [14]EtOH: Ethanol, [15]PanIN: pancreatic intraepithelial neoplasia

Simvastatin in Nanotechnology

The application of nanotechnology in parenteral drug delivery allowed researchers to overcome various challenges that conventional drug delivery systems could not resolve, such as nonspecific biodistribution and targeting, lack of water solubility, and poor oral bioavailability [44]. Furthermore, nanoparticles could be customized for size and surface characteristics to increase circulation time in the bloodstream and to maximize their delivery to the site of action without complications [45]. Nanoparticles were also found to readily penetrate tumors due to the tumors' discontinuous and leaky microvasculature [46] and accumulate at tumor site due to their poor lymphatic drainage that slows the clearance of the nanoparticles [47]. These structural features of many solid tumors are commonly referred to as the enhanced vascular permeability and retention (EPR) effect [48]. As a result, nanotechnologies have been used to overcome the challenges of the parenteral delivery of statins, mainly their limited aqueous solubility.

The need for a parenteral delivery system for simvastatin has been bolstered by the recent discoveries of its potential role in cancer therapy [49, 50]. When testing for its efficacy, however, simvastatin has mostly been given as an intraperitoneal injection of a low dose aqueous solution (Table 1). While simple and suitable for pre-clinical testing, such formulations may not be suitable for use in clinical studies. Therefore, techniques such as the entrapment of simvastatin in solid lipid nanoparticles and its dispersion in nanoemulsions have been developed and optimized as viable formulations for the parenteral administration of simvastatin. An overview of these technologies and a summary of the observed activity of simvastatin against tumor cells are provided in the following sections.

Nanostructured Lipid Carriers

Nanostructured lipid carriers (NLCs) are aqueous colloidal dispersions that range in size between 50 and 1000 nm [51]. The upper limit of this range is rarely approached as most NLCs do not exceed 300 nm [52-54]. The structure of NLCs is composed of blends of lipids in which liquid low melting-point lipids are entrapped in the form of oily nano-compartments within a solid lipid matrix [55]. NLCs could be readily prepared by high pressure homogenization, solvent emulsification/evaporation, and melt emulsification

[56-58] .While the melt emulsification method is frequently used, the quality of the NLCs prepared by this method could be diminished by the presence of larger particles in the range of micrometer, which may result in batch polydispersity. Therefore, ultrasound via probe sonicators is often employed to overcome this problem [59, 60] .

Melt emulsification with sonication technique was used by Ali et al. [61] to prepare simvastatin loaded NLCs, where sonication parameters, such as pulsar rate and sonication time, were optimized with the aid of a statistical model to attain submicron particles with high simvastatin entrapment efficiencies > 90% [62]. When preparing the NLCs, simvastatin is first solubilized in a lipid blend to form the core of the NLCs and then dispersed in an aqueous solution and stabilized with a suitable surfactant. To enhance the solubility of simvastatin in the lipid core of the NLCs and thereby increase its payload in the nanoparticles, secondary low melting point oil such as the tocotrienol-rich fraction (TRF) of palm oil is added to the lipid blend. Overall, the key elements to ensure the stability of the NLCs are the choice of the lipid blend and surfactant. Cetyl palmitate , Dynasan® 118, , Compritol® 888 ATO , and Precirol® ATO 5 are examples of high melting point lipids that are commonly used in the lipid blend for the preparation of NLCs [63] while Lutrol® F68 has been frequently used as the stabilizing surfactant [64, 65].

Decreasing the size of the NLCs could be readily achieved by decreasing lipid concentration in the dispersion and by increasing the surfactant to lipid ratio. To avoid bimodal particle size distribution due to an excess in the usage of surfactants, a compromise should be made on the appropriate amount of surfactant and lipids that would yield monomodal nanoparticles. A monomodal distribution is essential to allow for sterilization by filtration for subsequent use in parenteral and/or intravenous delivery [62]. For the simvastatin NLCs, optimal nanoparticles were obtained when NLC dispersions were made using a surfactant to lipid ratio of 0.5:1. For in vitro testing, a 1 mM simvastatin NLCs were prepared using Compritol® 888 ATO and TRF as the lipid phase (0.5%) and Lutrol® F68 (0.25%) as the stabilizer. The size of the nanoparticles was approximately 100 nm with a polydispersity index of 0.29±0.01, indicating that the nanoparticles were mono-disperse. The size of the nanoparticles was found to increase significantly when TRF was removed from the formulation. In general, the size of the NLCs may vary not only with the composition of each formulation but also with process parameters such as the difference in temperature between the warm microemulsion during preparation and storage conditions during the cooling process. These factors should be considered when scaling up to pilot studies. Another factor that should be monitored is the re-crystallization and precipitation of the entrapped drug from its solid solution or lipid dispersion. Therefore, the state of the disposition of simvastatin in the NLCs was investigated by differential scanning calorimetry (DSC) and powder X-ray diffraction (PXRD), which confirmed that simvastatin exists as a molecular dispersion in the TRF/lipid blend [61]. Entrapment of simvastatin in the NLCs was confirmed even after 6 months of storage by the absence of distinctive simvastatin endothermic peaks or crystalline pattern when analyzed by DSC and PXRD, respectively. To eliminate the possibility of drug expulsion from the nanoparticles during storage, NLC dispersions were visually inspected for signs of phase separation and were analyzed for simvastatin entrapment efficiency. No phase separation was observed and the percentage of simvastatin that remained entrapped in the nanoparticles after 6 months of storage remained > 90%.

In sink media composed of 30% ethanol in PBS buffer (pH 7.4), the release of simvastatin at 37°C from the NLCs was found to be biphasic. A burst period characterized by a fast simvastatin release was observed in the first 10 h followed by a slower and controlled release. Similar release pattern was reported for other NLCs where an initial fast release is followed by a slow and incomplete release of drug [66]. The cumulative percentage of simvastatin released over the 48 h test period was approximately 25%, which indicated that a large percentage of simvastatin was remained associated with the nanoparticles. While only a fraction of the drug was released into the media [61], the cytotoxicity of the formulations was not affected. This comes in agreement with several reports that showed that NLCs in which only a fraction of the drug is released are more cytotoxic than the free drug indicating that the cytotoxic compounds that remain associated with the nanoparticles are effective [66]. The slow and sustained release of simvastatin after the initial burst period also indicated that simvastatin was likely not present at or near the surface of the nanoparticles but instead within the cores of the NLCs as ideally predicted by the enhanced solvation ability of the nano-compartmental domains formed by the TRF.

The anticancer activity of the simvastatin NLCs was tested in vitro against neoplastic mammary epithelial cell line (+SA). The highly malignant +SA cells were derived from adenocarcinoma that developed spontaneously in BALB/c female mouse [67, 68]. They were shown to form adenocarcinoma that metastasize to the lungs when injected into the mammary gland fat pad of syngeneic female mice[67] and to exhibit the greatest degree of tumor progression or malignancy when compared with preneoplastic (CL-S1) and neoplastic (-SA) mouse mammary epithelial cells. Also tested was the contribution of TRF to the activity of the nanoparticles. TRF has an inherent antiproliferative activity against neoplastic +SA mammary epithelial cells. As with statins, TRF was shown to reduce HMGCoA reductase activity by causing post-transcriptional downregulation of the enzyme [69]. While the mechanism by which TRF and statins suppress HMGCoA reductase activity is different, a combined low dose treatment with γ-tocotrienol, a TRF isomer, and statins was shown to synergistically inhibit the growth of the highly malignant +SA mammary epithelial cells in culture [70]. Wali and Sylvester (2007) demonstrated that treatment with 0.25 μM simvastatin or 2.0 μM γ-tocotrienol alone had no effect, while the combined treatment with simvastatin and γ-tocotrienol significantly inhibited the proliferation of malignant +SA mammary epithelial cells. Combining low dose of statin and tocotrienol was shown to induce mammary tumor cell cycle arrest at Gap phase 1 (G1), resulting from an increase in p27 expression, and a corresponding decrease in cyclin D1, CDK2, and hypophosphorylation of Rb protein [71]. Therefore combining TRF with simvastatin in NLCs may prove not only effective in delivering the required therapeutic concentration of simvastatin to the tumor cells but also minimize non-specific toxicity resulting from its systemic administration.

The activity of simvastatin in NLCs and the synergistic effect of TRF was confirmed by Ali et al., [61] who examined the in vitro antiproliferative effects of simvastatin and TRF when combined and co-encapsulated within the cores of the lipid nanoparticles against the highly malignant +SA mammary epithelial cells. The half maximal inhibitory concentration (IC50) value of blank NLCs loaded with TRF alone was 1.5 μM, which decreased 3 folds to 0.52 μM when simvastatin was added to the NLCs at a simvastatin to TRF ratio of 1:5. These results confirmed the cytotoxic effect of simvastatin and the potential therapeutic benefits of a combined simvastatin and TRF treatment.

Parenteral Lipid Emulsions

Parenteral Lipid Emulsions are dispersions of immiscible liquids (usually oil and water), in which the oil droplets are dispersed in the water phase and stabilized by a surfactant [72]. They have been used for over 50 years in medical applications as a source of calories for patients who require parenteral feeding and to prevent or reverse fatty acid deficiency [73, 74]. The exact composition of these emulsions has changed over the years. Initially, oils used in lipid emulsions consisted of digestible long-chain triglycerides (LCT), such as soybean oil [75]. The impairment in the function of the clotting and immunological systems [76] and the increase in lipid peroxidation in vivo [77] as a consequence to the infusion of LCTs, however, led to the development of a second generation of lipid emulsions. In these emulsions the LCT was partially substituted with medium-chain triglycerides (MCT), which have a faster rate of hydrolysis by lipoprotein lipase (LpL) leading to more rapid clearance [78, 79]. Emulsion with a 1:1 MCT:LCT blend have also been used in Europe, Asia, and South America to avoid "linoleic acid overload'', a condition caused by excessive quantity (52–54%) of linoleic acid (C18:2 ω-6), and ω-6 polyunsaturated fatty acid (PUFA) in soybean oil [80, 81]. More recently, a third-generation has been developed in which oils with biological activity, such as fish oil, olive oil and purified palm oil, have been used to contribute to the therapeutic value of these emulsions [82, 83].

Overall, parenteral emulsions are biodegradable, they are physically stable, and are widely regarded as safe and often less toxic than other formulations due to the natural source of their components [84]. Lecithin or phospholipids derived from soybean egg yolk, for example, are often used as the surfactant to prevent the phase separation in emulsions. The biocompatibility of formulations intended for intravenous delivery is particularly critical for the safety of patients [85, 86]. Therefore, the in vitro assessment of the hemolytic effect of parenteral lipid emulsions is considered a reliable measure for estimating membrane damage caused by the formulation when given in vivo [87]. In a study by Alayoubi et al. [88], parenteral emulsions stabilized with sodium oleate and sodium deoxycholate, for example, were found to induce hemolysis, which significantly increased with time. Emulsions stabilized with sodium oleate and sodium deoxycholate were also found to be sensitive to electrolytes and exhibited poor physical stability. On the other hand, emulsions PEGylated with high concentrations of Poloxamer® 188 or DSPE-PEG(2000) did not induce significant hemolytic effect [89]. They were also found to be stable in the presence of electrolytes and under physical stress. Stability of these emulsions was attributed to the surface decoration with bulky polyoxyethylene head groups that made it difficult for the droplets to approach the erythrocytes, thereby reducing direct contact between the phospholipids and cell membrane [87, 90, 91]. The use of steric stabilizers was also shown to produce stable formulations [92].

In addition to their safety, parenteral lipid emulsions could be readily manufactured on a large scale [93], which makes them more attractive over the other intravenous delivery systems. [94]. High pressure homogenization technique, in particular, has been widely used in the pharmaceutical industry to manufacture parenteral lipid emulsions [95]. The intense shear, cavitation, and turbulent flow in the narrow valves of the homogenizer during the emulsification process [96] leads to the reduction in droplet size of the emulsion and the deflocculation of the clusters of primary fat globules [97]. Therefore, critical process parameters such as the number of homogenization cycles and homogenization pressure are often optimized during manufacturing [98, 99]. Poor processing of the emulsions may produce extra stress on emulsion droplets leading to their destabilization.

Due to their numerous advantages, parenteral lipid emulsions have been explored as a delivery vehicle for drugs with poor aqueous solubility [100]. Because of their oil core and capacity to solubilize drugs, lipid emulsions were also considered for the parenteral delivery of simvastatin. Recently Alayoubi et al. [101] developed a lipid emulsion with high simvastatin load by using a mixture of vitamin E and MCT as the oil phase of the emulsions. MCT was primarily added to lower the viscosity of vitamin E, which was used to aid in the solubilization of simvastatin and to enhance its therapeutic effect. During preliminary screening and process optimization it was found that high pressures and repeated homogenization was needed to process emulsions made with high vitamin E content. As a result, the Vitamin/MCT ratio was found to be the most significant contributor to the stability of these emulsions [88]. Poor stability was observed when the percentage of vitamin E in the blend exceeded 70% [102]. Eventually, in the optimized formulation, simvastatin was incorporated into the emulsion at a loading of 9% w/w of the oil phase with 100% entrapment efficiency.

The droplet size of the simvastatin emulsion was 224±2 nm with a polydispersity index of 0.115 ± 0.028 and a zeta potential of 45 ± 1 mV [101]. Polydispersity index typically ranges from 0, to indicate a monodisperse system, to 0.5, indicating a relatively broad distribution [103]. Emulsions with narrow droplet size distribution are required as evident by the low polydispersity index of commercial parenteral lipid emulsions such as Intralipid®. Stability of parenteral lipid emulsions is also highly correlated with zeta potential. It was reported that zeta potential values below −30 mV impart sufficient electrostatic repulsion between the nanoparticles, which favor improved physical stability [104]. As to their morphology the droplets of the emulsion were spherical, near-spherical and ellipsoidal when visualized by Scanning Transmission Electron Microscopy (STEM). No crystals or drug precipitation was detected when samples were inspected by polarized light microscopy.

No significant ($p > 0.05$) change in droplet size of the simvastatin emulsion was observed after 6 months of storage in refrigerated conditions (4-8°C) and after 48 h of incubation in culture media at 37°C, which simulate the conditions during the in vitro antiproliferation studies. Moreover, no change in either peak intensity or shift in elusion time was noticed when the oxidation and/or degradation of simvastatin was monitored by HPLC over 6 months of storage, which confirmed the chemical stability of simvastatin in the emulsion. Although no oxidation or degradation products were observed, additional stability studies under elevated temperature and different light intensities should be considered when developing emulsion for clinical use.

The release of simvastatin from the emulsion was also monitored in simulated body fluid that mimics the electrolyte chemistry of blood [105]. A biphasic release profile was observed where an initial fast release during the first 6 h was followed by a phase of slower and controlled release. After 48 h, only approximately 20% of simvastatin was released. Similar low cumulative drug release was reported for other nanoparticles formulations [66, 106]. It indicates that simvastatin was more likely to be disposed within the core rather than the surface of the emulsion. The viscosity of the oil phase might have also played a role in delaying the diffusion of simvastatin from the emulsion.

The activity of the simvastatin emulsions was subsequently tested [101]. As discussed earlier, the anticancer activity of simvastatin entrapped in NLCs was demonstrated against the highly malignant murine +SA mammary tumor cells [107]. For more clinical relevance, the activity of simvastatin emulsion was tested against human mammary tumor epithelial MCF-7 and MDA-MB-231 cells. MCF7 are estrogen-receptor (ER) positive whereas the MDA-MB-231 cells are ER negative [108]. In addition, MDA cells express constitutively higher levels of epidermal growth factor receptor (EGFR) and protein Kinase C (PKC) activity [108, 109], which are common targets for many anticancer drugs [110].

The IC50 values of simvastatin when used alone were 19 and 8 μM against MCF-7 and MDA-MB-231 cells, respectively. A significant improvement in activity was observed when simvastatin was formulated into a lipid emulsion with an IC50 of 10.3 and 4.9 μM against MCF-7 and MDA-MB-231 cells, respectively. It is worth noting that the IC50 value of simvastatin, if given alone, is significantly higher than the concentration of simvastatin that has been used in the simvastatin emulsion, which ranged from 0.04 to 2.2 μM. Due to the low solubility of simvastatin in the oil phase of the emulsions, the maximum molar ratio between simvastatin and vitamin E that could be attained was 1:11. Nevertheless, even at these low levels of simvastatin loading, a significant increase in the potency of the emulsion was observed, which was in agreement with those previously observed with +SA cells [106].

Conclusion

Studies, both in vitro and in vivo have confirmed the anticancer activity of simvastatin and demonstrated its potential use in cancer therapy and/or prevention. Higher doses of simvastatin, however, are needed to exert these effects in vivo. Delivering simvastatin at therapeutic levels presents a challenge due to the poor aqueous solubility of statins. Therefore, while many studies have tested the activity of simvastatin after oral administration; very few have evaluated the potential therapeutic benefits of the parenteral administration of simvastatin. To circumvent these challenges, specialized drug delivery systems have been developed to safely deliver high loads of simvastatin though the parenteral routes of administration. Lipid based drug delivery systems, such as lipid emulsions and solid lipid nanocarriers or nanostructured lipid carriers represent two promising approaches for the delivery of simvastatin. In addition to their physical stability and ease of manufacture, preliminary studies in vitro have demonstrated that entrapment of simvastatin is such carriers not only retains but also enhances its anticancer activity. Studies have also suggested that further potentiation in the anticancer activity of simvastatin may be attained by the co administration of other drug or molecules, such as tocotrienols, that act synergistically to suppress tumor growth. Further studies are needed to test the efficacy of these delivery systems in the clinic.

References

[1] Graaf, MR; Richel, DJ; van Noorden, CJ; Guchelaar, HJ. Effects of statins and farnesyltransferase inhibitors on the development and progression of cancer. *Cancer Treat Rev.*, 2004, 30(7), 609-41.

[2] Habenicht, AJ; Glomset, JA; Ross, R. Relation of cholesterol and mevalonic acid to the cell cycle in smooth muscle and swiss 3T3 cells stimulated to divide by platelet-derived growth factor. *J Biol Chem.*, 1980, 255(11), 5134-40.

[3] Fairbanks, KP; Witte, LD; Goodman, DS. Relationship between mevalonate and mitogenesis in human fibroblasts stimulated with platelet-derived growth factor. *J Biol Chem.*, 1984, 259(3), 1546-51.

[4] Kaneko, I; Hazama-Shimada, Y; Endo, A. Inhibitory effects on lipid metabolism in cultured cells of ML-236B, a potent inhibitor of 3-hydroxy-3-methylglutaryl-coenzyme-A reductase. *Eur J Biochem/FEBS.* 1978, 87(2), 313-21.

[5] Quesney-Huneeus, V; Galick, HA; Siperstein, MD; Erickson, SK; Spencer, TA; Nelson, JA. The dual role of mevalonate in the cell cycle. *J Biol Chem.*, 1983, 258(1), 378-85.

[6] Campbell, MJ; Esserman, LJ; Zhou, Y; Shoemaker, M; Lobo, M; Borman, E; et al. Breast cancer growth prevention by statins. *Cancer Res.*, 2006, 66(17), 8707-14.

[7] Seeger, H; Wallwiener, D; Mueck, AO. Statins can inhibit proliferation of human breast cancer cells in vitro. *Exp Clin Endocr Diab.*, 2003, 111(1), 47-8.

[8] Shibata, MA; Ito, Y; Morimoto, J; Otsuki, Y. Lovastatin inhibits tumor growth and lung metastasis in mouse mammary carcinoma model: a p53-independent mitochondrial-mediated apoptotic mechanism. *Carcinogenesis.*, 2004, 25(10), 1887-98.

[9] Denoyelle, C; Vasse, M; Korner, M; Mishal, Z; Ganne, F; Vannier, JP; et al. Cerivastatin, an inhibitor of HMG-CoA reductase, inhibits the signaling pathways involved in the invasiveness and metastatic properties of highly invasive breast cancer cell lines: an in vitro study. *Carcinogenesis.*, 2001, 22(8), 1139-48.

[10] Demierre, MF; Higgins, PD; Gruber, SB; Hawk, E; Lippman, SM., Statins and cancer prevention. *Nat Rev Cancer.*, 2005, 5(12), 930-42.

[11] Kusama, T; Mukai, M; Iwasaki, T; Tatsuta, M; Matsumoto, Y; Akedo, H; et al. Inhibition of epidermal growth factor-induced RhoA translocation and invasion of human pancreatic cancer cells by 3-hydroxy-3-methylglutaryl-coenzyme a reductase inhibitors. *Cancer res.*, 2001, 61(12), 4885-91.

[12] Malliri, A; Collard, JG. Role of Rho-family proteins in cell adhesion and cancer. *Curr Opin Cell Biol.*, 2003, 15(5), 583-9.

[13] Mazieres, J; Tillement, V; Allal, C; Clanet, C; Bobin, L; Chen, Z; et al. Geranylgeranylated, but not farnesylated, RhoB suppresses Ras transformation of NIH-3T3 cells. *Exp Cell Res.*, 2005, 304(2), 354-64.

[14] Simpson, KJ; Dugan, AS; Mercurio, AM. Functional analysis of the contribution of RhoA and RhoC GTPases to invasive breast carcinoma. *Cancer res.*, 2004, 64(23), 8694-701.

[15] Zugaza, JL; Caloca, MJ; Bustelo, XR. Inverted signaling hierarchy between RAS and RAC in T-lymphocytes. *Oncogene.*, 2004, 23(34), 5823-33.

[16] Ghosh-Choudhury, N; Mandal, CC; Ghosh-Choudhury, N; Ghosh, Choudhury, G. Simvastatin induces derepression of PTEN expression via NFkappaB to inhibit breast cancer cell growth. *Cell Signal.*, 2010, 22(5), 749-58.

[17] Kucharczak, J; Simmons, MJ; Fan, Y; Gelinas, C. To be, or not to be: NF-kappaB is the answer--role of Rel/NF-kappaB in the regulation of apoptosis. *Oncogene.*, 2003, 22(56), 8961-82.

[18] Micheau, O; Tschopp, J. Induction of TNF receptor I-mediated apoptosis via two sequential signaling complexes. *Cell.*, 2003, 114(2), 181-90.

[19] Fang, LW; Tai, TS; Yu, WN; Liao, F; Lai, MZ., Phosphatidylinositide 3-kinase priming couples c-FLIP to T cell activation. *J Biol Chem.*, 2004, 279(1), 13-8.

[20] Luo, JL; Kamata, H; Karin, M. IKK/NF-kappaB signaling: balancing life and death--a new approach to cancer therapy. *J Clin Invest.*, 2005, 115(10), 2625-32.

[21] Hanahan, D; Weinberg, RA., The hallmarks of cancer. *Cell.*, 2000, 100(1), 57-70.

[22] Vousden, KH; Lu, X. Live or let die: the cell's response to p53. *Nat Rev Cancer.*, 2002, 2(8), 594-604.

[23] Chipuk, JE; Green, DR. Dissecting p53-dependent apoptosis. *Cell Death Differ.*, 2006, 13(6), 994-1002.

[24] Vaseva, AV; Moll, UM. The mitochondrial p53 pathway. *Biochim Biophys Acta.*, 2009, 1787(5), 414-20.

[25] Huang, S; Pettaway, CA; Uehara, H; Bucana, CD; Fidler, IJ. Blockade of NF-kappaB activity in human prostate cancer cells is associated with suppression of angiogenesis, invasion, and metastasis. *Oncogene.*, 2001, 20(31), 4188-97.

[26] Kiriakidis, S; Andreakos, E; Monaco, C; Foxwell, B; Feldmann, M; Paleolog, E. VEGF expression in human macrophages is NF-kappaB-dependent: studies using adenoviruses expressing the endogenous NF-kappaB inhibitor IkappaBalpha and a kinase-defective form of the IkappaB kinase 2. *J Cell Sci.*, 2003, 116(Pt 4), 665-74.

[27] Fujioka, S; Niu, J; Schmidt, C; Sclabas, GM; Peng, B; Uwagawa, T, et al. NF-kappaB and AP-1 connection: mechanism of NF-kappaB-dependent regulation of AP-1 activity. *Mol Cell Biol.*, 2004, 24(17), 7806-19.

[28] Karin, M; Yamamoto, Y; Wang, QM. The IKK NF-kappa B system: a treasure trove for drug development. *Nat Rev Drug Discov.*, 2004, 3(1), 17-26.

[29] Greten, FR; Eckmann, L; Greten, TF; Park, JM; Li, ZW; Egan, LJ; et al. IKKbeta links inflammation and tumorigenesis in a mouse model of colitis-associated cancer. *Cell.*, 2004, 118(3), 285-96.

[30] McIntyre, BS; Briski, KP; Gapor, A. Sylvester PW. Antiproliferative and apoptotic effects of tocopherols and tocotrienols on preneoplastic and neoplastic mouse mammary epithelial cells. *Proceedings of the Society for Experimental Biology and Medicine Society for Experimental Biology and Medicine.*, 2000, 224(4), 292-301.

[31] McIntyre, BS; Briski, KP; Tirmenstein, MA; Fariss, MW; Gapor, A; Sylvester, PW. Antiproliferative and apoptotic effects of tocopherols and tocotrienols on normal mouse mammary epithelial cells. *Lipids.*, 2000, 35(2), 171-80.

[32] Allen, L; Allen, LV; Ansel, HC. Ansel's Pharmaceutical Dosage Forms and Drug Delivery Systems: Wolters Kluwer Health, 2013.

[33] Hatefi, A; Amsden, B., Biodegradable injectable in situ forming drug delivery systems. *J Control Release.*, 2002, 80(1-3), 9-28.

[34] Mownika, G; Srinivas, P. Formulation and evaluation of simvastatin injectable in situ implants. *Am J Drug Discov Dev.*, 2012, 2, 87-100.

[35] Kochuparambil, ST; Al-Husein, B; Goc, A; Soliman, S; Somanath, PR. Anticancer efficacy of simvastatin on prostate cancer cells and tumor xenografts is associated with inhibition of Akt and reduced prostate-specific antigen expression. *J Pharmacol Exp Ther.*, 2011, 336(2), 496-505.

[36] Manu, KA; Shanmugam, MK; Li, F; Chen, L; Siveen, KS; Ahn, KS; et al. Simvastatin sensitizes human gastric cancer xenograft in nude mice to capecitabine by suppressing nuclear factor-kappa B-regulated gene products. *J Mol Med.*, 2014, 92(3), 267-76.

[37] Mandal, CC; Ghosh-Choudhury, N; Yoneda, T; Choudhury, GG; Ghosh-Choudhury, N. Simvastatin prevents skeletal metastasis of breast cancer by an antagonistic interplay between p53 and CD44. *J Biol Chem.*, 2011, 286(13), 11314-27.

[38] Zanfardino, M; Spampanato, C; De, Cicco, R; Buommino, E; De, Filippis, A; Baiano, S; et al. Simvastatin reduces melanoma progression in a murine model. *Int J Oncol.*, 2013, 43(6), 1763-70.

[39] Goc, A; Kochuparambil, ST; Al-Husein, B; Al-Azayzih, A; Mohammad, S; Somanath, PR. Simultaneous modulation of the intrinsic and extrinsic pathways by simvastatin in mediating prostate cancer cell apoptosis. *BMC cancer.*, 2012, 12, 409.

[40] Clutterbuck, RD; Millar, BC; Powles, RL; Newman, A; Catovsky, D; Jarman, M; et al. Inhibitory effect of simvastatin on the proliferation of human myeloid leukaemia cells in severe combined immunodeficient (SCID) mice. *Brit J Haematol.*, 1998, 102(2), 522-7.

[41] Lee, J; Lee, I; Han, B; Park, JO; Jang, J; Park, C; et al. Effect of simvastatin on cetuximab resistance in human colorectal cancer with KRAS mutations. *J Natl Cancer I.*, 2011, 103(8), 674-88.

[42] Lee, SJ; Lee, I; Lee, J; Park, C; Kang, WK. Statins, 3-hydroxy-3-methylglutaryl coenzyme A reductase inhibitors, potentiate the anti-angiogenic effects of bevacizumab by suppressing angiopoietin2, BiP, and Hsp90alpha in human colorectal cancer. *Brit J Cancer.*, 2014, 111(3), 497-505.

[43] Fendrich, V; Sparn, M; Lauth, M; Knoop, R; Plassmeier, L; Bartsch, DK; et al. Simvastatin delay progression of pancreatic intraepithelial neoplasia and cancer formation in a genetically engineered mouse model of pancreatic cancer. *Pancreatology.*, 2013, 13(5), 502-7.

[44] Cho, K; Wang, X; Nie, S; Chen, ZG; Shin, DM. Therapeutic nanoparticles for drug delivery in cancer. *Clin Cancer Res.*, 2008, 14(5), 1310-6.

[45] Zhang, XQ; Xu, X; Bertrand, N; Pridgen, E; Swami, A; Farokhzad, OC. Interactions of nanomaterials and biological systems: Implications to personalized nanomedicine. *Adv Drug Deliver Rev.*, 2012, 64(13), 1363-84.

[46] Hobbs, SK; Monsky, WL; Yuan, F; Roberts, WG; Griffith, L; Torchilin, VP, et al. Regulation of transport pathways in tumor vessels: role of tumor type and microenvironment. *Proceedings of the National Academy of Sciences.*, 1998, 95(8), 4607-12.

[47] Moghimi, SM; Hunter, AC; Murray, JC. Long-circulating and target-specific nanoparticles: theory to practice. *Pharmacol Rev.*, 2001, 53(2), 283-318.

[48] Maeda, H; Wu, J; Sawa, T; Matsumura, Y; Hori, K. Tumor vascular permeability and the EPR effect in macromolecular therapeutics: a review. *J Control Release.*, 2000, 65(1), 271-84.
[49] Cho, SJ; Kim, JS; Kim, JM; Lee, JY; Jung, HC; Song, IS. Simvastatin induces apoptosis in human colon cancer cells and in tumor xenografts, and attenuates colitis-associated colon cancer in mice. *Int J Cancer.*, 2008, 123(4), 951-7.
[50] Koyuturk, M; Ersoz, M; Altiok, N. Simvastatin induces apoptosis in human breast cancer cells: p53 and estrogen receptor independent pathway requiring signalling through JNK. *Cancer Lett.*, 2007, 250(2), 220-8.
[51] Khalil, RM; Abd-Elbary, A; Kassem, MA; Ghorab, MM; Basha, M., Nanostructured lipid carriers (NLCs) versus solid lipid nanoparticles (SLNs) for topical delivery of meloxicam. *Pharm Dev Technol.*, 2013, 19(3), 304-14.
[52] Patel, D; Dasgupta, S; Dey, S; Ramani, YR; Ray, S; Mazumder, B. Nanostructured lipid carriers (NLC)-based gel for the topical delivery of aceclofenac: preparation, characterization, and in vivo evaluation. *Scientia pharmaceutica.*, 2012, 80(3), 749.
[53] How, CW; Abdullah, R; Abbasalipourkabir, R. Physicochemical properties of nanostructured lipid carriers as colloidal carrier system stabilized with polysorbate 20 and polysorbate 80. *Afr J Biotechnol.*, 2013, 10(9), 1684-9.
[54] Loo, CH; Basri, M; Ismail, R; Lau, HLN; Tejo, BA; Kanthimathi, M; et al. Effect of compositions in nanostructured lipid carriers (NLC) on skin hydration and occlusion. *Int J Nanomed.*, 2013, 8, 13.
[55] Jenning, V; Mäder, K; Gohla, SH. Solid lipid nanoparticles (SLN) based on binary mixtures of liquid and solid lipids: a (1) H-NMR study. *Int J Pharm.*, 2000, 205(1-2), 15-21.
[56] Feng, F; Zheng, D; Zhang, D; Duan, C; Wang, Y; Jia, L; et al. Preparation, characterization and biodistribution of nanostructured lipid carriers for parenteral delivery of bifendate. *J Microencapsul.*, 2011, 28(4), 280-5.
[57] Varshosaz, J; Eskandari, S; Tabbakhian, M. Freeze-drying of nanostructure lipid carriers by different carbohydrate polymers used as cryoprotectants. *Carbohyd Polym.*, 2012, 88(4), 1157-63.
[58] Shangguan, M; Lu, Y; Qi, J; Han, J; Tian, Z; Xie, Y; et al. Binary lipids-based nanostructured lipid carriers for improved oral bioavailability of silymarin. *J Biomater Appl.*, 2014, 28(6), 887-96.

[59] Lin, X; Li, X; Zheng, L; Yu, L; Zhang, Q; Liu, W. Preparation and characterization of monocaprate nanostructured lipid carriers. *Colloid Surface A.*, 2007, 311(1-3), 106-11.

[60] Huang, G; Zhang, N; Bi, X; Dou, M. Solid lipid nanoparticles of temozolomide: potential reduction of cardial and nephric toxicity. *Int J Pharm.*, 2008, 355(1), 314-20.

[61] Ali, H; Shirode, AB; Sylvester, PW; Nazzal, S. Preparation, characterization, and anticancer effects of simvastatin–tocotrienol lipid nanoparticles. *Int J Pharm.*, 2010, 389(1), 223-31.

[62] Ali, H; Shirode, AB; Sylvester, PW; Nazzal, S. Preparation and *in vitro* antiproliferative effect of tocotrienol loaded lipid nanoparticles. Colloid Surface A., 2010, 353(1), 43-51.

[63] Das, S; Chaudhury, A. Recent advances in lipid nanoparticle formulations with solid matrix for oral drug delivery. *AAPS PharmSciTech.*, 2011, 12(1), 62-76.

[64] Araujo, J; Gonzalez-Mira, E; Egea, M; Garcia, M; Souto, E. Optimization and physicochemical characterization of a triamcinolone acetonide-loaded NLC for ocular antiangiogenic applications. *Int J Pharm.*, 2010, 393(1), 168-76.

[65] Puglia, C; Offerta, A; Rizza, L; Zingale, G; Bonina, F; Ronsisvalle, S., Optimization of curcumin loaded lipid nanoparticles formulated using High Shear Homogenization (HSH) and Ultrasonication (US) methods. *J Nanosci Nanotechno.*, 2013, 13(10), 6888-93.

[66] Wong, HL; Bendayan, R; Rauth, AM; Li, Y; Wu, XY., Chemotherapy with anticancer drugs encapsulated in solid lipid nanoparticles. *Adv Drug Deliver Rev.*, 2007, 59(6), 491-504.

[67] Anderson, L; Danielson, K; Hosick, H. Epithelial cell line and subline established from premalignant mouse mammary tissue. *In Vitro.* 1979, 15(11), 841-3.

[68] Danielson, KG; Anderson, LW; Hosick, HL. Selection and Characterization in Culture of Mammary Tumor Cells with Distinctive Growth Properties in Vivo. *Cancer Res.*, 1980, 40(6), 1812-9.

[69] McIntyre, BS; Briski, KP; Gapor, A; Sylvester, PW. Antiproliferative and apoptotic effects of tocopherols and tocotrienols on preneoplastic and neoplastic mouse mammary epithelial cells. *Proceedings of the Society for Experimental Biology and Medicine.*, 2000, 224(4), 292-301.

[70] Wali, VB; Sylvester, PW. Synergistic antiproliferative effects of γ-tocotrienol and statin treatment on mammary tumor cells. *Lipids.*, 2007, 42(12), 1113-23.

[71] Wali, VB; Bachawal, SV; Sylvester, PW. Combined treatment of γ-tocotrienol with statins induce mammary tumor cell cycle arrest in G1. *Exp Biol Med.*, 2009, 234(6), 639-50.
[72] Waitzberg, DL; Torrinhas, RS; Jacintho, TM. New parenteral lipid emulsions for clinical use. *JPEN J Parenter Enteral Nutr.*, 2006, 30(4), 351-67.
[73] Cukier, C; Waitzberg, DL; Logullo, AF; Bacchi, CE; Travassos, VH; Torrinhas, RS; et al. Lipid and lipid-free total parenteral nutrition, differential effects on macrophage phagocytosis in rats. *Nutrition.*, 1999, 15(11-12), 885-9. Epub 1999/11/27.
[74] Uncles, DR. Intravenous lipid emulsions in anaesthesia. *BMJ.*, 2011, 342.
[75] Von, Corswant, C; Thorén, P; Engström, S. Triglyceride-based microemulsion for intravenous administration of sparingly soluble substances. *J Pharm Sci.*, 1998, 87(2), 200-8.
[76] Manuel-y-Keenoy; L, Nonneman; Bosscher, HD; Vertommen, J; Schrans, S; Klu¨tsch, K; et al. Effects of intravenous supplementation with atocopherol in patients receiving total parenteral nutrition containing medium- and long-chain triglycerides. *Eur J Clin Nutr.*, 2002, 56(2), 121–8.
[77] Wu, GH; Jarstrand, C; Nordenstrom, J. Phagocyte-induced lipid peroxidation of different intravenous fat emulsions and counteractive effect of vitamin E. *Nutrition.*, 1999, 15(5), 359-64. Epub 1999/06/04.
[78] Lai, HS; Lin, WH; Wu, HC; Chang, KJ; Chen, WJ. Effects of a medium-chain triacylglycerol/long-chain triacylglycerol fat emulsion containing a reduced ratio of phospholipid to triacylglycerol in pediatric surgical patients. *Nutrition.*, 2005, 21(7-8), 825-30. Epub 2005/06/25.
[79] Deckelbaum, RJ; Hamilton, JA; Moser, A; Bengtsson-Olivecrona, G; Butbul, E; Carpentier, YA; et al. Medium-chain vs long-chain triacylglycerol emulsion hydrolysis by lipoprotein lipase and hepatic lipase: implications for the mechanisms of lipase action. *Biochemistry.*, 1990, 29(5), 1136-42.
[80] Deckelbaum, RJa; Calder, PCb; Carpentier, YAc. Using different intravenous lipids: underutilized therapeutic approaches? [Miscellaneous]. *Curr Opin Clin Nutr.*, 2004, 7(2), 113-5.
[81] Ton, MN; Chang, C; Carpentier, YA; Deckelbaum, RJ. In vivo and in vitro properties of an intravenous lipid emulsion containing only medium chain and fish oil triglycerides. *Clin Nutr.*, 2005, 24(4), 492-501.

[82] Hartman, C; Ben-Artzi, E; Berkowitz, D; Elhasid, R; Lajterer, N; Postovski, S; et al. Olive oil-based intravenous lipid emulsion in pediatric patients undergoing bone marrow transplantation: a short-term prospective controlled trial. *Clin Nutr.*, 2009, 28(6), 631-5. Epub 2009/06/06.

[83] Goulet, O; Antebi, H; Wolf, C; Talbotec, C; Alcindor, LG; Corriol, O; et al. A new intravenous fat emulsion containing soybean oil, medium-chain triglycerides, olive oil, and fish oil: a single-center, double-blind randomized study on efficacy and safety in pediatric patients receiving home parenteral nutrition. *JPEN J Parenter Enteral Nutr.*, 2010, 34(5), 485-95. Epub 2010/09/21.

[84] Hippalgaonkar, K; Majumdar, S; Kansara, V. Injectable lipid emulsions-advancements, opportunities and challenges. *AAPS PharmSciTech.*, 2010, 11(4), 1526-40. Epub 2010/10/27.

[85] Banziger, R. Hemolysis testing in vivo of parenteral formulations. *Bull Parenter Drug Assoc.* 1967, 21(4), 148-51. Epub 1967/07/01.

[86] Doenicke, A; Roizen, MF; Nebauer, AE; Kugler, A; Hoernecke, R; Beger-Hintzen, H. A comparison of two formulations for etomidate, 2-hydroxypropyl-beta-cyclodextrin (HPCD) and propylene glycol. *Anesth Analg.*, 1994, 79(5), 933-9. Epub 1994/11/01.

[87] Jumaa, M; Kleinebudde, P; Müller, BW., Physicochemical properties and hemolytic effect of different lipid emulsion formulations using a mixture of emulsifiers. *Pharm Acta Helv.*, 1999, 73(6), 293-301.

[88] Alayoubi, A; Kanthala, S; Satyanarayanajois, SD; Anderson, JF; Sylvester, PW; Nazzal, S. Stability and in vitro antiproliferative activity of bioactive "Vitamin E" fortified parenteral lipid emulsions. *Colloid Surface B.*, 2013, 103, 23-30.

[89] Alayoubi, A; Alqahtani, S; Kaddoumi, A; Nazzal, S. Effect of PEG surface conformation on anticancer activity and blood circulation of nanoemulsions loaded with tocotrienol-rich fraction of palm oil. *The AAPS journal.*, 2013, 15(4), 1168-79.

[90] Forster, D; Washington, C; Davis, SS. Toxicity of Solubilized and Colloidal Amphotericin B Formulations to Human Erythrocytes. *J Pharm Pharmacol.*, 1988, 40(5), 325-8.

[91] Weingarten, C; Santos, Magalhaes, NS; Baszkin, A; Benita, S; Seiller, M. Interactions of a non-ionic ABA copolymer surfactant with phospholipid monolayers: Possible relevance to emulsion stabilization. *Int J Pharm.*, 1991, 75(2-3), 171-9.

[92] Heurtault, B; Saulnier, P; Pech, B; Venier-Julienne, M-C; Proust, J-E; Phan-Tan-Luu, R; et al. The influence of lipid nanocapsule composition on their size distribution. *Eur J Pharm Sci.*, 2003, 18(1), 55-61.

[93] Li, J; Nie, S; Yang, X; Wang, C; Cui, S; Pan, W. Optimization of tocol emulsions for the intravenous delivery of clarithromycin. *Int J Pharm.*, 2008, 356(1-2), 282-90.

[94] Constantinides, PP; Tustian, A; Kessler, DR. Tocol emulsions for drug solubilization and parenteral delivery. *Adv Drug Deliver Rev.*, 2004, 56(9), 1243-55.

[95] Lamprecht, A; Ubrich, N; Hombreiro, Perez, M; Lehr, C; Hoffman, M; Maincent, P. Biodegradable monodispersed nanoparticles prepared by pressure homogenization-emulsification. *Int J Pharm.*, 1999, 184(1), 97-105. Epub 1999/07/30.

[96] Desrumaux, A; Marcand, J. Formation of sunflower oil emulsions stabilized by whey proteins with high-pressure homogenization (up to 350 MPa), effect of pressure on emulsion characteristics. *Int J Food Sci Tech.*, 2002, 37(3), 263-9.

[97] Floury, J; Desrumaux, A; Lardières, J. Effect of high-pressure homogenization on droplet size distributions and rheological properties of model oil-in-water emulsions. *Innov Food Sci Emerg.*, 2000, 1(2), 127-34.

[98] Jumaa, M; Müller, BW. The effect of oil components and homogenization conditions on the physicochemical properties and stability of parenteral fat emulsions. *Int J Pharm.*, 1998, 163(1-2), 81-9.

[99] Barnadas-Rodriguez, R; Sabes, M., Factors involved in the production of liposomes with a high-pressure homogenizer. Int J Pharm., 2001, 213(1-2), 175-86. Epub 2001/02/13.

[100] Jumaa, M; Müller, BW., Parenteral emulsions stabilized with a mixture of phospholipids and PEG-660-12-hydroxy-stearate: evaluation of accelerated and long-term stability. *Eur J Pharm Biopharm.*, 2002, 54(2), 207-12.

[101] Alayoubi, AY; Anderson, JF; Satyanarayanajois, SD; Sylvester, PW; Nazzal, S. Concurrent delivery of tocotrienols and simvastatin by lipid nanoemulsions potentiates their antitumor activity against human mammary adenocarcenoma cells. *Eur J Pharm Sci.*, 2013, 48(3), 385-92.

[102] Alayoubi, A; Nazzal, M; Sylvester, PW; Nazzal, S., "Vitamin E" fortified parenteral lipid emulsions: Plackett-Burman screening of primary process and composition parameters. *Drug Dev Ind Pharm.*, 2013, 39(2), 363-73.

[103] Cheong, JN; Tan, CP; Man, YBC; Misran, M. α-Tocopherol nanodispersions: Preparation, characterization and stability evaluation. *J Food Eng*., 2008, 89(2), 204-9.

[104] Freitas, C; Müller, RH. Effect of light and temperature on zeta potential and physical stability in solid lipid nanoparticle (SLN™) dispersions. *Int J Pharm*., 1998, 168(2), 221-9.

[105] Marques, MRC; Loebenberg, R; Almukainzi, M. Simulated Biological Fluids with Possible Application in Dissolution Testing. *Dissolution Technologies*., 2011, 18(3), 15-28.

[106] Ali, H; Shirode, AB; Sylvester, PW; Nazzal, S. Preparation, characterization, and anticancer effects of simvastatin–tocotrienol lipid nanoparticles. *Int J Pharm*., 2010, 389(1–2), 223-31.

[107] Wali, V; Sylvester, P. Synergistic Antiproliferative Effects of γ-Tocotrienol and Statin Treatment on Mammary Tumor Cells. *Lipids*., 2007, 42(12), 1113-23.

[108] Lacroix, M; Haibe-Kains, B; Hennuy, BJF; Laes, F; Lallemand, I. Gonze; et al. Gene regulation by phorbol 12-myristate 13-acetate in MCF-7 and MDA-MB-231, two breast cancer cell lines exhibiting highly different phenotypes. *Oncol Rep*., 2004, 12(4), 701-7.

[109] Wang, K; Wang, K; Li, W; Huang, T; Li, R; Wang, D; et al. Characterizing breast cancer xenograft epidermal growth factor receptor expression by using near-infrared optical imaging. *Acta Radiol*., 2009 50(10), 1095—103

[110] Aggarwal, BB; Sundaram, C; Prasad, S; Kannappan, R. Tocotrienols, the vitamin E of the 21st century: its potential against cancer and other chronic diseases. *Biochem Pharmacol*., 2010, 80(11), 1613-31. Epub 2010/08/11.

Index

B

C

D

E

F

G

J

K

L

M

N

O

P

Q

R

S

T

U

V

W

X

Y

Z